HEALTHY
SPEEDY
SUPPERS

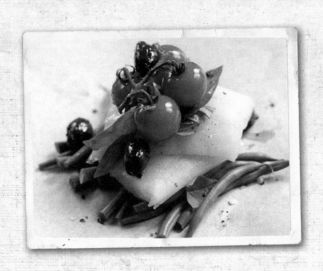

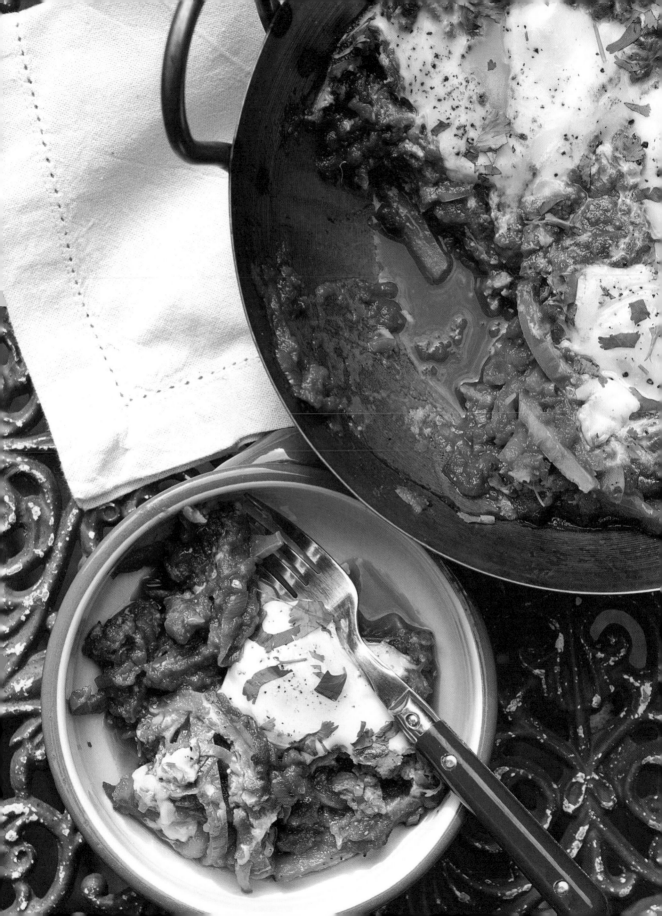

KATRIONA MACGREGOR

HEALTHY SPEEDY SUPPERS

*Quick, nutritious and delicious
recipes for busy people*

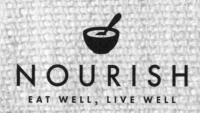

NOURISH
EAT WELL, LIVE WELL

To my foodie parents and Grandmum;
all serious cooks who got me started in the kitchen.

Healthy Speedy Suppers
Katriona MacGregor

First published in the UK and USA in 2016 by
Nourish, an imprint of Watkins Media Limited
19 Cecil Court
London WC2N 4EZ

enquiries@nourishbooks.com

Managing Editor: Rebecca Woods
Editor: Becky Alexander
Design Manager: Viki Ottewill
Designer: Geoff Borin
Production: Uzma Taj

A CIP record for this book is available from the
British Library

ISBN: 978-1-84899-299-3

10 9 8 7 6 5 4 3 2 1

Typeset in Trade Gothic and Bradley Hand
Colour reproduction by XY Digital
Printed in China

Publisher's note:
While every care has been taken in compiling the
recipes for this book, Watkins Media Limited, or any
other persons who have been involved in working on this
publication, cannot accept responsibility for any errors
or omissions, inadvertent or not, that may be found in
the recipes or text, nor for any problems that may arise
as a result of preparing one of these recipes. If you are
pregnant or breastfeeding or have any special dietary
requirements or medical conditions, it is advisable to
consult a medical professional before following any
of the recipes contained in this book.

Notes:
Unless otherwise stated:
• Use medium eggs, fruit and vegetables
• Use fresh ingredients, including herbs and spices
• Do not mix imperial and metric measurements
• 1 teaspoon = 5ml 1 tablespoon = 15ml 1 cup = 240ml

nourishbooks.com

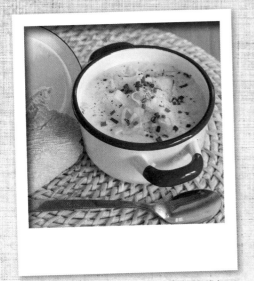

CONTENTS

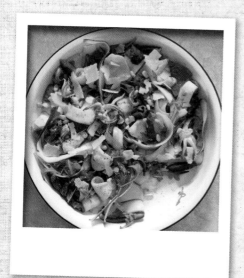

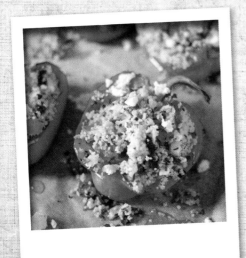

HEALTHY EATING FOR THE TIME POOR

*My Speedy Weeknight Suppers column in the **Telegraph** came about after a shameful slump in my diet following a return to London office life. Despite being a trained cook and fully-fledged food obsessive, I found myself returning home exhausted, my love of wholesome eating and good ingredients lost to the convenience of ready meals and boiled eggs with soldiers; a state of affairs that left me tired and unsatisfied.*

Being a lifetime lover of flavours and fresh ingredients, I decided to take action, and the result was a collection of weekly supper recipes that are quick and easy to prepare, healthy, nutritious and affordable, often leaving something for lunch the next day. Each recipe has been put to the test at home after a busy day in the office; with the ingredients usually scooped up on the way home. The ingredient lists are as short as possible and the methods relaxed, often one-dish cooking. After a couple of years of devising weeknight recipes, it seemed the right time to bring the recipes together in this book, featuring old favourites alongside some new.

MAKING NEW CHOICES

Having been diagnosed with a thyroid condition in 2014, I began to learn about the importance of diet in treating this disease, which affects millions of people worldwide. While my recipes had always been light and appetizing, the focus changed to include less wheat, cows' milk,

fat, refined carbohydrates and sugar, all of which can play havoc with auto-immune disease sufferers. The role of diet and eating well is incredibly compelling when it comes to health. For me, it's about including a wide variety of freshly cooked foods, especially vegetables, in your daily meals; this has made a tremendous difference to how I feel over a surprisingly short time.

Cooking without some of our Western staples opened my eyes to a huge array of new flavours, ingredients and cooking methods, and showed me that you can cook delicious, satisfying food without a reliance on wheat and dairy. Take, for instance, the Chicken and Sweetcorn Broth (see page 20) which I would have previously made with wheat-based noodles, and now use rice noodles. The Quinoa, Courgette and Herb Cakes (see page 160) use quinoa and cornflour/ cornstarch to bind them, rather than breadcrumbs and flour. A lot of the Indian-inspired recipes include coconut milk or no dairy at all, with the option to serve yogurt alongside rather than as an ingredient.

Many people include diary and wheat in their diet without any problem at all, and I do still use these ingredients, but where possible I use gluten- and

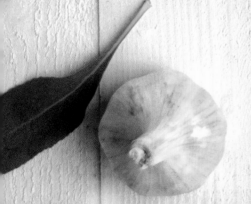
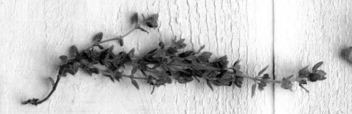

dairy-free alternatives such as Japanese tamari sauce in place of Chinese soy sauce. I wanted to give people the option and to explain how easy these tweaks are to make in your daily cooking. Even if you don't have an intolerance, it can be good to include new ingredients in your diet for variety. Of course, swapping the highly processed carbohydrates in your diet for wholewheat pasta and bread, and wholegrain or wild rice is a good idea for anyone; in any case, these ingredients have much more flavour and texture than the white alternatives. The Mushroom and Wild Rice Pilaf (see page 146) would only be a shadow of what it should be if made with white rice rather than the lovely combination of red, wild and brown grains I suggest.

THINKING ABOUT SHOPPING

We're lucky to live in a country with an abundance of food at our fingertips and a huge range of international ingredients available, yet too often we rely on the offering of our nearest supermarket. While it's almost impossible in the chaos of modern living to avoid supermarkets completely, it makes sense to me to use them for dry supplies and staples, leaving the fresh ingredients to be bought on the day you need them from local suppliers or markets. This way you're more likely to be able to support local food producers while making sure what you're buying is fresh and tasty. Locally bought, seasonal and, if possible, organic vegetables have far more nutritional value than the supermarket equivalent which has been ripened in transit, packaged in plastic and kept chilled in crates for weeks. You'll also find yourself avoiding a fridge full of ingredients bought in bulk that end up being thrown away once they've passed their sell-by date.

SPEEDY COOKING AND PLANNING AHEAD

All of the recipes take less than 40 minutes to cook, with many taking as little as 15 or 20 minutes. Each recipe is labelled with a time flash so you can see at a glance how long you have until your supper's ready. Asian soups and stir-fries are particularly quick, as are the raw salads, pasta and fish dishes. Doubling the recipe quantities is a great way to save time and stress during the week. Making a dish for eight people takes little more time than for four and means you have another meal for later in the week, or lunches to take to work. Many of the recipes also freeze well, especially the soups, curries and casseroles, so if you're only cooking for one or two you can easily stock up on frozen meals for time-pressed moments. Cheaper, tastier and, of course, a lot healthier than a mass-made, supermarket-bought ready meal.

I'm still surprised by how often people mention they're fearful when it comes to cooking fish; in fact, fish is the ultimate fast food, taking no time at all to cook. Take, for instance, the recipe for Cod, Green Bean and Cherry Tomato Parcels (see page 110) or the Sea Bass with Thai Vegetables (see page 108); both are super-simple as well as light and healthy.

The first part of this book is dedicated to stocking your larder and acquiring some basic staples so that you're able to make meals without lengthy shopping lists. Once you have those building blocks in the cupboard, you're most of the way there. The aim of this book is for you to be able to cook simple dishes with ease and confidence, without the obstacles that might leave you reaching for a ready meal. If you have some spices, an onion or two and some canned tomatoes already at home, all you need is some fresh chicken and a curry is born.

For me, the most important thing is to enjoy cooking and to celebrate not only the wonderful ingredients we are lucky enough to have available to us but also the delight of eating. It's a joy to cook and eat together and to nourish yourself and your family with healthful, seasonal recipes that have the power to make you feel healthy, well and energized.

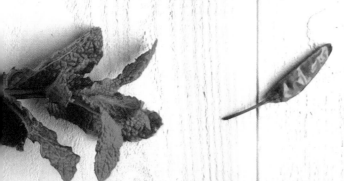

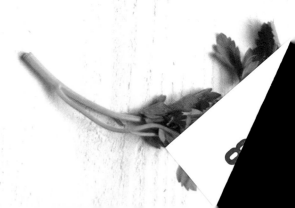

LARDER ESSENTIALS

Food shopping should be more of a pleasure than it often is in our busy modern lives. There is so much satisfaction to be had from shopping locally, talking to suppliers and buying fresh, seasonal produce that you have seen, smelt and chosen. For most of us though, after a long day at work, food shopping is, more often than not, a time-pressed chore.

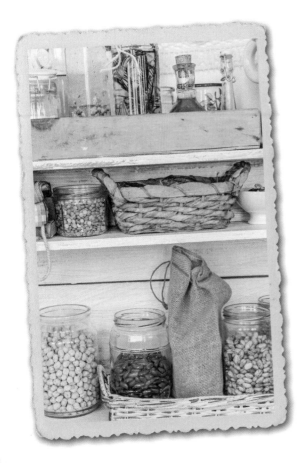

Keeping a cupboard or two full of staple ingredients means that, for me, during the week I can simply add a few fresh ingredients to the seasonings, dry stores or jarred ingredients that I've got at home, making mid-week shopping and cooking much more manageable. If you're lucky enough to work near local shops, this might even mean you can nip out to a good butcher or fishmonger at lunchtime and pick up something delicious without having to brave a supermarket queue.

I'm not suggesting you rush out and buy everything on this list, but having a few long-lasting ingredients – pulses, tomatoes, spices and seasonings, a jar or two of mustard and some oils and vinegars – to hand, will make pulling together a delicious supper much simpler.

There are also a few kitchen tools I've had with me in all of my kitchens, no matter how little space there is, which I'd recommend anyone has to keep things as quick and as easy as possible.

NOTE: With all food, buy the best quality that you can afford, organic where possible and if you can afford it, especially when it comes to fresh meat, dairy, eggs and vegetables. If the expense of organic means you eat less of these ingredients, that's no bad thing – an organically produced foodstuff will be packed with far more nutrients than its conventionally produced equivalent.

OILS AND VINEGARS

You don't need a huge array of these to get started but a few bottles will arm you for most of the recipes in this book.

OILS

Keeping a small selection of different oils is a great idea so that you can easily create a versatile selection of dishes. The most important distinction is between oils you use for cooking and oils you use for dressings and drizzling. Rapeseed/canola oil, sunflower oil and coconut oil are great for general cooking, having higher smoke points. Extra virgin olive oil, and oils from nuts and seeds, are better used in dressings and for drizzling over or flavouring dishes that have already been cooked. This isn't set in stone though; if I were roasting Mediterranean vegetables, I'd still use olive oil, but not extra virgin. If you're using butter to fry with, add a little rapeseed/canola or sunflower oil to the pan to prevent the milk solids from burning.

VINEGARS

Having a varied selection of vinegar is useful for last-minute dressings and flavourings, with certain kinds lending themselves particularly well to specific dishes or regional cuisines. Red wine vinegar is slightly sweet and makes a more mellow dressing than white, while balsamic is not only good for sweet dressings but also as a seasoning for Mediterranean tomato-based sauces.

It's also delicious reduced down to a thick, sticky glaze – as in the recipe for Fig, Prosciutto and Gorgonzola Croutes (see page 86) – which you can keep in a jar to drizzle over all sorts of finished dishes and salads. Sherry vinegar has a lovely, winey depth and adds interest to a basic vinaigrette, while Japanese rice vinegar, which has a mild flavour, is great for vegetable and fish dishes.

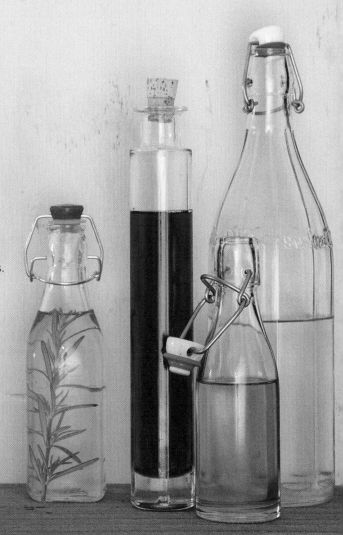

SEASONINGS

To add flavour to your dishes, keep a small range of seasonings, herbs and spices to hand. The variety available in the supermarket is staggering, but the selection you can store at home is probably limited by space.

SEA SALT AND BLACK PEPPER

The most basic seasonings, essential for bringing out flavour in your dishes. Freshly ground black pepper is always preferable, so invest in a decent pepper mill. I tend to use run-of-the-mill pouring table salt during cooking, keeping a box of lovely bright white sea salt flakes to sprinkle onto finished dishes.

DRIED HERBS

While there is no replacement for fresh herbs when it comes to salads and sauces – for example in Salsa Verde (see page 94) and Classic Pesto (see page 170) – dried herbs are great for soups, stews, casseroles and curries. I always have jars of dried oregano, thyme, bay leaves, dill and rosemary in the cupboard. For these, as well as dried spices below, it's much more economical to buy large packets from the world food aisles or from a market rather than the tiny jars more commonly purchased. Dried herbs and spices can lose their flavour and go stale if they're not used, so keep them in carefully sealed containers and replace them if you've had them for a long time.

DRIED SPICES

The selection of dried spices available can be quite intimidating and a bit of an unknown entity to a new cook, but they're worth exploring as they're incredibly versatile, can quickly add flavour to dishes and have many residual health benefits. Having a jar

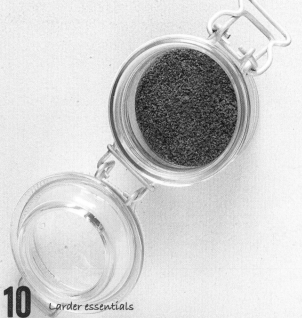
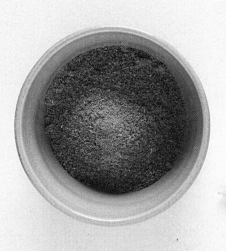

of garam masala to hand, for instance, can be a last minute lifesaver, meaning a simple curry is only a few ingredients away. I would suggest gradually building up a stock of the following spices: paprika and smoked paprika, turmeric, chilli powder, ground coriander, ginger, garam masala, ground cumin, black and yellow mustard seeds, fennel seeds and, my favourite, nigella (black onion) seeds. Apart from having a stock of spices for cooking, you'll have everything you need for delicious marinades as well.

SAUCES AND MUSTARDS

Staples in my kitchen are soy sauce (I use tamari soy sauce because it is gluten-free and I prefer the slightly less intensely salty flavour) and Worcestershire sauce, which is very useful as a seasoning, giving depth to lamb dishes or lifting rich cheese dishes such as Welsh Rarebit. Fish sauce, Tabasco and sweet chilli sauce are also useful to have to hand. My kitchen would be bereft without a selection of mustards, which add so much to all sorts of dishes – from dressings to sauces, and from casseroles to a plate of steak and chips. Wholegrain, Dijon and English mustard are the essential starting points, but the hotter varieties are worth experimenting with, too.

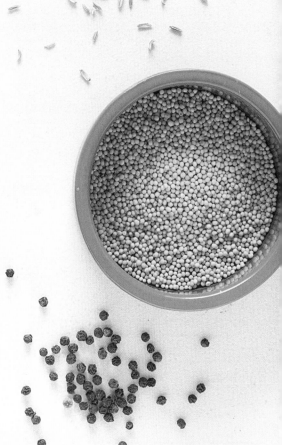

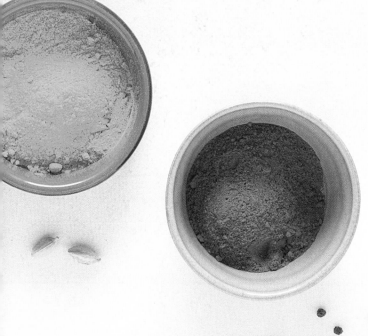

DRY STORES

Heavy to carry home and heavy on space, these are definitely ingredients to try to plan ahead with, and perhaps add to an online order every month or so.

PASTA AND NOODLES

A variety of pasta and noodles are handy to keep in stock for time-pressed evenings, both needing very little cooking time. They can easily be rustled up into a delicious feast without a huge amount of fuss, as in the recipe for Spicy Prawn and Tomato Spaghetti (page 122). As well as spaghetti, a packet of linguine and a variety of your favourite pasta shapes – mine being conchiglie and penne – are useful to have stashed away for emergencies. For stir-fries, Asian soups and even salads, some rice and/or egg noodles are a good basic staple, too. Since I made substantial changes to my diet over the last two years, I always use gluten-free pasta and noodles of which there are now many good varieties, especially in larger wholefood shops.

GRAINS AND PULSES

For risottos and pilafs or simply as an accompaniment, basmati, wild and Arborio rice are the basics. But there is a wonderful selection of interesting varieties available to us now, offering different textures and tastes, such as beautiful French red Camargue (used in the Mushroom and Wild Rice Pilaf on page 146), fragrant jasmine or nutty brown rice. Other grains I make regular use of are quinoa, couscous and bulgur wheat – all quick to cook, versatile grains that lend well to salads and side dishes. For those avoiding wheat or gluten, couscous and bulgur wheat are to be avoided; quinoa makes a great alternative.

Beans and pulses in cans or packets, such as lentils, chickpeas, kidney beans, butter/lima beans and cannellini can be used as the main ingredient in dishes such as Chickpea and Black-eyed Bean Chilli (page 136) or Chorizo, Leek and Cider-Braised Lentils (page 84). They're also a good way to make casseroles and curries go a little bit further, being inexpensive but very nutritious and filling. And for anyone with a dip addiction such as mine, a can of chickpeas or butter/lima beans can be whizzed up into a delicious homemade hummus for a last-minute dip or sandwich filling with very little work.

PRESERVED VEGETABLES

Apart from the canned pulses already mentioned, canned tomatoes, tomato purée/paste, olives, anchovies, capers and sun-dried tomatoes are ingredients you'll find cropping up frequently throughout this book. This isn't only because I'm a fan of Mediterranean flavours with their natural depth of flavour and satisfying piquancy, but also because these ingredients will last for what seems like forever in cans and jars at the back of a cupboard. Just when you think there really isn't anything to make supper with, a can of tomatoes will usually appear, which along with some onions, capers and olives can become a delicious sauce for chicken, pasta or fish (see Chicken Puttanesca on page 62). The Italians are experts at bottling and preserving, managing to pack a huge amount of flavour into their canned tomatoes and bottled passata; a pair of ingredients worth spending a little more money on to avoid the sometimes bitter acridness of the cheaper brands, to which you may find yourself having to add sugar.

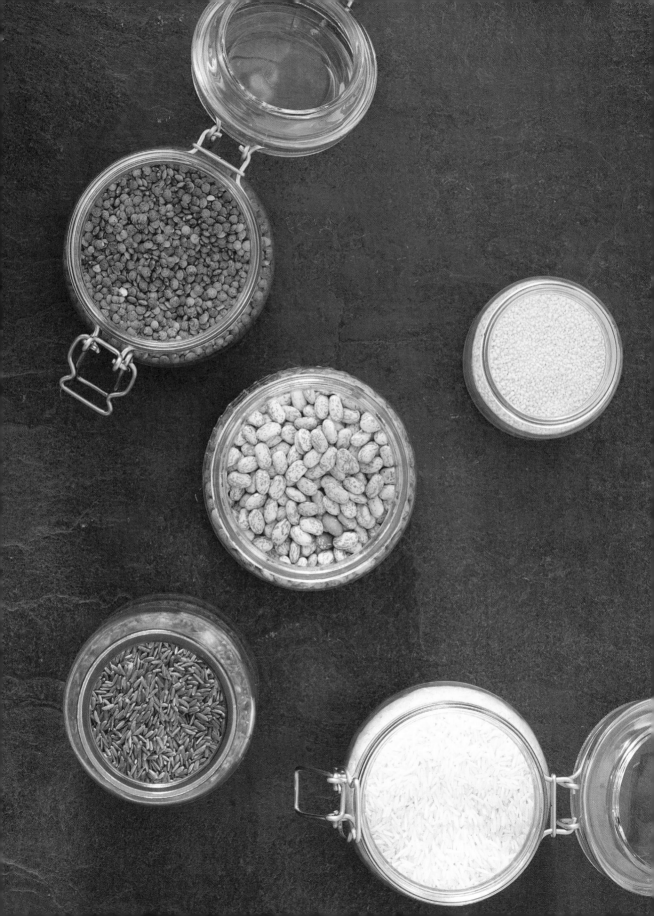

NUTS AND SEEDS

Pine nuts for pesto or salads are a staple, and definitely better if you take the time to toast them to a rich golden brown before use. A packet of cashews, walnuts, almonds or pistachios are wonderful to have to hand to add texture to salads or pilafs, while at the same time adding nutrients – they're a great source of protein and fat and are satiating as well as flavoursome. Pumpkin and sesame seeds, too, are similarly useful and, like nuts, benefit from being toasted before use.

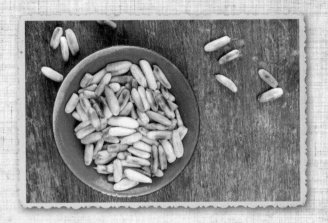

DELICIOUS EXTRAS

For a food lover the list could go on and on, especially with the rich variety of ingredients we have access to nowadays. Limited though by space and time, I try not to keep filling my cupboards each time I spy something new or exciting, instead trying to decide what to cook based on what I already have. Apart from those already mentioned, I wouldn't be without a jar of runny honey for making salad dressings and marinades; coconut milk and tamarind paste for curries; tom yum paste for Thai soups and the best-quality chicken or vegetable bouillon (stock) you can find. Oh, and a pack of crispy fried shallots to sprinkle on top of anything I can persuade myself might need them; they are absolutely one of the most moreish ingredients around.

FRESH, FRIDGE & FREEZER

Finally, a few fresh and frozen ingredients that are worth buying regularly, allowing you to whip up a soup, side dish or omelette with very little thought.

FRESH

Onions, garlic, chillies, ginger, carrots, celery, parsley, new potatoes and leeks.

FRIDGE

Eggs, butter, goats' cheese, cooking chorizo and Parmesan cheese.

FREEZER

Peas, sweetcorn and broad/fava beans, good-quality chicken stock and uncooked prawns/shrimp.

ESSENTIAL TOOLS

I wouldn't be without anything on this list, particularly the pans and knives. Some of them may sound painfully obvious but there are a lot of kitchens I've arrived in to cook that have been without.

KNIVES AND A SHARPENER

Kitchen kit where you can really break the bank! If you're considering buying knives, go for quality rather than quantity. A few well-made kitchen knives in sizes that you find comfortable to use will definitely change your attitude to cooking; you only really need three: a good-sized cook's knife, a smaller one of a similar shape, and a serrated knife for slicing, and you'll be able to survive. There's nothing worse, though, than a blunt knife, so definitely buy yourself a sharpener or make friends with your butcher who will probably sharpen them for you free of charge if you're a regular customer.

PANS, DISHES AND OVENWARE

In the long run you'll save money if you invest in well-made pans rather than cheap basics. A wide, heavy based frying pan, a couple of decent lidded saucepans, a casserole dish and a few oven sheets will get you started. As a general rule when you're choosing, the heavier the pan the better; the lightweight, non-stick options won't last and will warp and lose their shape.

OTHER ESSENTIALS

A sharp grater (I use a Microplane), julienne peeler, potato peeler, a mini food processor, hand-held blender, tongs with rubber edges, wooden spoons, a couple of spatulas, scales and a colander are all, without doubt, worth investing in.

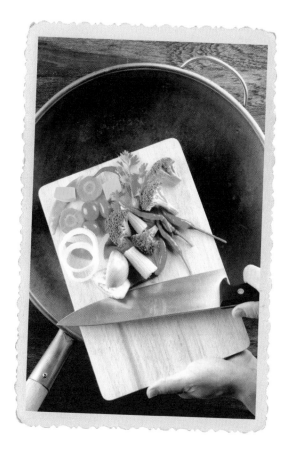

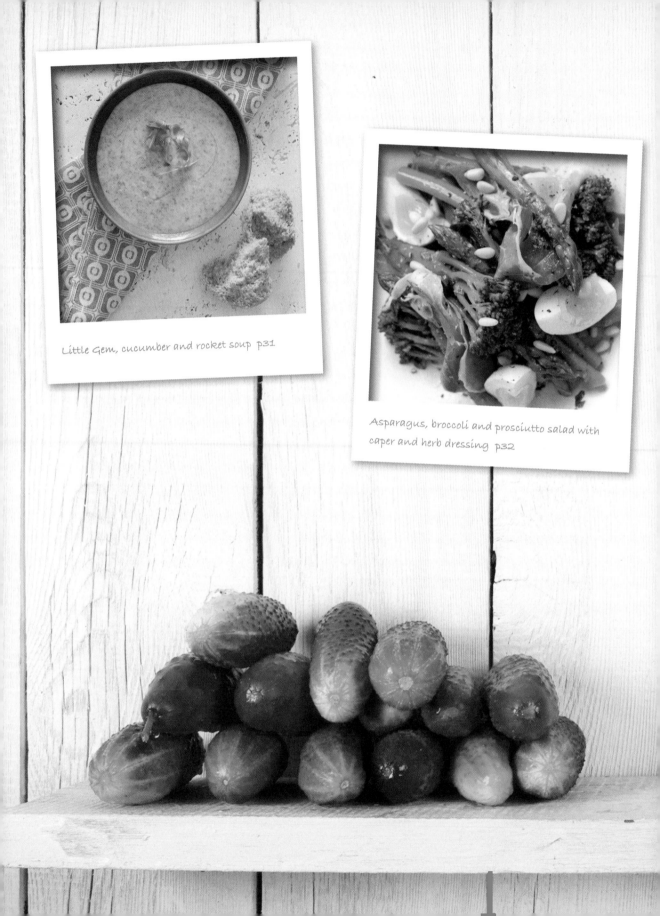

Little Gem, cucumber and rocket soup p31

Asparagus, broccoli and prosciutto salad with caper and herb dressing p32

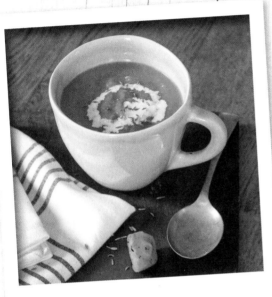

Roast carrot, tomato and dill soup p26

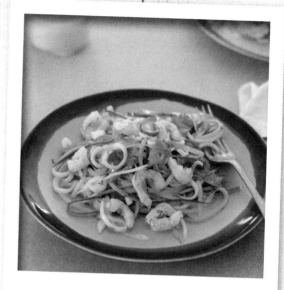

Prawn, courgette and coriander salad p43

SOUPS & SALADS

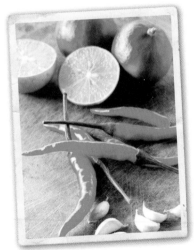

SPICY BEEF AND NOODLE BROTH

This is one of those staples that once in your repertoire will appear on the table again and again, both because of its ease to make and its delicious aromatic flavours. I can't think of many dishes more nourishing than a bowl of rich, stocky noodles with fresh herbs and spices.

READY IN **15** MINUTES

SERVES 4

300g/10½oz dried noodles (rice, egg or udon)

1l/35fl oz/4 cups beef stock

1 garlic clove, finely chopped

5cm/2in piece of root ginger, peeled and grated

1 red chilli, deseeded and finely chopped

bunch of spring onions/ scallions, sliced

1 star anise

juice of 1 lime

2 tbsp soy sauce

1 tsp fish sauce

pinch of brown sugar

2 handfuls of coriander/ cilantro leaves, chopped

300g/10½oz rump steak, sliced into thin strips

¼ red pepper, shredded

handful of bean sprouts

lime wedges, to serve

Bring a pan of water to the boil and cook the noodles according to the package directions. Drain and leave to one side.

Meanwhile, pour the stock into a large pan and bring to the boil. Add the garlic, ginger, chilli, spring onions/scallions and star anise to the stock. Simmer for 5 minutes.

Squeeze the juice of the lime into the soup followed by the soy sauce, fish sauce, brown sugar and half of the coriander/cilantro leaves. Simmer for 2 minutes before tasting to check the seasoning; add a little more soy sauce or sugar if either are needed.

Drop the steak into the broth, bring back to a simmer, then remove the pan from the heat. Leave to rest for a couple of minutes.

Pile the noodles into deep bowls and ladle the soup over the top, discarding the star anise. Sprinkle with the red pepper, bean sprouts and the remaining coriander/cilantro leaves, and serve with wedges of lime, for squeezing.

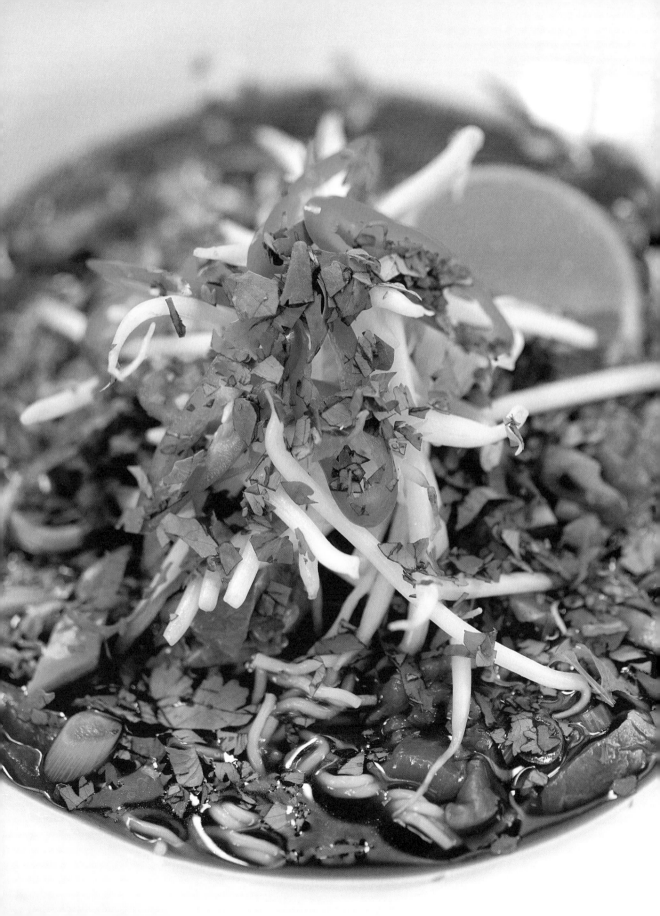

CHICKEN AND SWEETCORN BROTH

SERVES 4

READY IN
15
MINUTES

2l/70fl oz/8½ cups
chicken stock

2 sweetcorn cobs

1 large courgette/zucchini,
finely diced

1 leek, finely sliced into rounds

2 handfuls of parsley, finely
chopped, plus extra for sprinkling

2 nests of dried vermicelli
rice noodles

225g/8oz cooked chicken,
shredded

freshly ground black pepper

single/light cream, to serve
(optional)

An old-fashioned kitchen classic, this recipe reminds me of gathering round a family table on a wet, wintry day and being warmed through by the nourishing flavours. Being a simple, clear soup, it relies on a really good stock, ideally made at home from chicken bones that remain from a Sunday roast. Failing that, a good deli- or butcher-bought tub of fresh stock will suffice, but avoid cubes, which won't give you the same depth of flavour.

Pour the stock into a large saucepan and bring to the boil. Turn down to a gentle simmer.

Use a sharp knife to slice the kernels from the sweetcorn cobs. Tip into the simmering stock along with the courgette/zucchini and leek. Bring back to the boil then simmer gently for 8–10 minutes until the sweetcorn is tender.

Add the parsley, rice noodles and chicken and simmer for another 2–3 minutes until the noodles are tender.

Season with plenty of black pepper and ladle into deep bowls. Sprinkle with a little more chopped parsley, or if you like, a swirl of cream.

TOM YUM, PRAWN AND MUSHROOM SOUP

With Thai ingredients so readily available now, I'd love you to try this recipe, which uses one of the brilliant soup pastes you can buy. While a home-made paste makes a world of difference to a fragrant curry, a good-quality shop-bought paste is ideal for a quick soup, and it saves a lot of time chopping.

Begin by pouring the stock into a large saucepan, then add the tom yum paste, ginger and lemongrass. Bring to the boil and tip in the spring onions/scallions, mushrooms and sweetcorn. Simmer for 5 minutes before adding the prawns/shrimp.

Bring back to a gentle simmer and cook for 1–2 minutes until the prawns/shrimp have turned pink and opaque. Stir in the coconut milk, soy sauce, fish sauce and lime juice and bring back almost to a simmer, being careful not to boil the soup.

Throw in the coriander/cilantro leaves and serve the soup in deep bowls.

READY IN
15
MINUTES

SERVES 4

700ml/24fl oz/3 cups vegetable stock

4 tbsp tom yum paste

2cm/¾in piece of root ginger, peeled and sliced

1 lemongrass stalk, sliced

4–6 spring onions/scallions, sliced

115g/4oz mushrooms, sliced

115g/4oz baby sweetcorn, sliced

400g/14oz raw peeled king prawns/jumbo shrimp

400ml/14fl oz/1⅔ cups coconut milk

1 tbsp soy sauce

1 tbsp fish sauce

juice of 1 lime

handful of coriander/cilantro leaves

SMOKED HADDOCK AND LEEK CHOWDER

Smoky and creamy, this soup warms you from the inside out. If you prefer a smooth consistency you can blend the soup before adding the flaked smoked haddock at the end of the recipe.

SERVES 4

400g/14oz smoked haddock fillets

1 bay leaf

a few peppercorns

600ml/21fl oz/2½ cups semi-skimmed/low-fat milk

50g/1¾oz/¼ cup butter

2 leeks, finely sliced

2 large potatoes (about 400g/14oz), peeled and cubed

400ml/14fl oz/1⅔ cups vegetable stock

1 heaped tsp Dijon mustard

170ml/5½fl oz/⅔ cup double/heavy cream

juice of ½ lemon

small handful of parsley, roughly chopped

sea salt and freshly ground black pepper

handful of chives, chopped, for sprinkling

crusty bread, to serve

Place the smoked haddock in a shallow pan with the bay leaf and peppercorns and pour over the milk. Bring gently to the boil and simmer over a very low heat for 2 minutes until the haddock is just cooked through. Lift the haddock out of the pan with a slotted spoon and leave both the fish and milk to one side.

Melt the butter in a deep saucepan and add the leeks. Cook for 2–3 minutes until they've begun to wilt and soften, then add the potatoes. Cover with a lid and cook gently for 10 minutes, stirring occasionally to stop the vegetables sticking.

Add the reserved milk to the vegetables, followed by the stock. Bring to the boil and simmer for 5 minutes, then stir in the mustard and add a good grind of black pepper.

Gently flake the haddock with your fingers into small pieces, discarding any bones you find. Tip the fish into the soup, followed by the cream, lemon juice and parsley. Stir well and return the pan to the heat to heat through; make sure it's piping hot but be careful not to let the soup boil.

Taste to check the seasoning, adding more mustard, lemon or black pepper if you think it needs it. Scatter over the chives and serve with crusty bread.

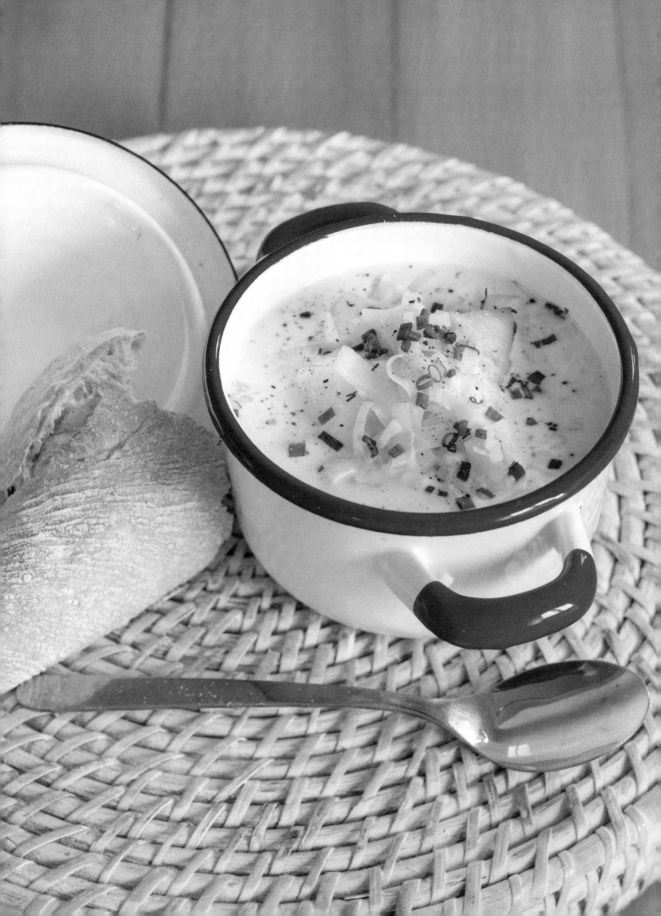

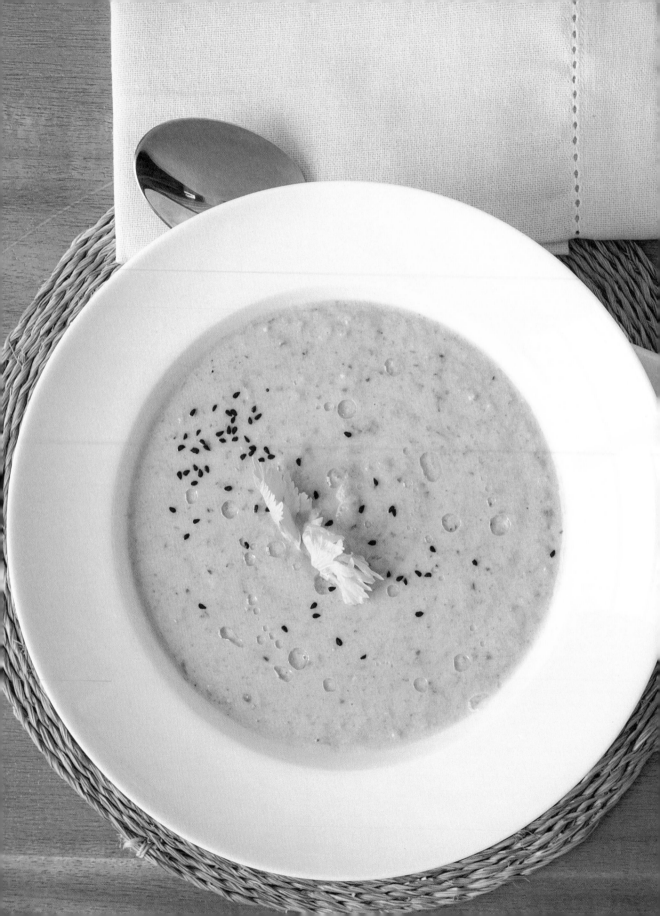

CELERY AND WALNUT SOUP

As the cold starts to creep in under the kitchen door, there's nothing more warming to come home to than a steaming bowl of soup. With toasted walnuts, a little cream and the sweetness of a leek, this recipe tastes a lot more sophisticated than it really is.

Preheat the oven to 190°C/375°F/gas 5.

Spread the walnuts on a baking sheet and place in the middle of the oven for 8–10 minutes, or until just golden. Put in a blender and whizz to coarse crumbs or chop as finely as you can with a knife.

Meanwhile, wash the celery and chop finely, discarding the stringy outer stalks, roots and ends. Keep a few leaves for serving.

Melt the butter in a large saucepan and heat until just beginning to sizzle. Add the chopped onion, leek, celery and garlic and cook gently, covered with a lid, for 10 minutes, stirring occasionally. Tip in the nigella seeds, potato and parsley and cook for a minute longer. Pour in the stock and bring to the boil. Turn down to a simmer and cook for 10–15 minutes until the potato and celery are soft and easily crushed with the back of a fork.

Season with salt and pepper before adding the cream. Pour into a blender or use a hand-held blender to blend to a smooth, velvety consistency. Then add the walnuts and a squeeze of lemon juice and blend briefly to combine.

Serve with extra nigella seeds or walnuts scattered over the top, a drizzle of walnut oil if you have it, a few celery leaves and lots of warm bread.

SERVES 4

110g/4oz/¾ cup walnut halves, plus extra to serve (optional)

5 celery stalks

50g/1¾oz/¼ cup butter

½ onion, peeled and chopped

1 leek, sliced

1 garlic clove, peeled and crushed

½ tsp nigella (black onion) seeds, plus extra to serve

1 large potato (about 200g/7oz), peeled and diced

handful of parsley, chopped

800ml/28fl oz/3¼ cups chicken stock

100ml/3½fl oz/scant ½ cup double/ heavy cream

squeeze of lemon juice

sea salt and freshly ground black pepper

walnut oil, to serve (optional)

crusty bread, to serve

NOTE: With pale white stems and sweet, nutty flavour, Fenland celery is a wonderful seasonal ingredient to make the most of in winter months. Grown with rich Fenland soil banked up over its bulbs as a protective blanket from frosty weather, it keeps a clean crunch ideal for salads or crudités.

ROAST CARROT, TOMATO AND DILL SOUP

Roasting the carrots and onions imparts a deep, caramelized flavour to this soup. Like a French potage it is thick, filling and warming; lovely served in generous mugs. Oh, and it is incredibly simple to make.

SERVES 4

READY IN 40 MINUTES

500g/1lb 2oz carrots, chopped into bite-size pieces

2 onions, sliced

2 garlic cloves

2 tbsp olive oil

400g/14oz/1¾ cups canned chopped tomatoes

100g/3½oz/¾ cup dried red lentils

handful of dill

1 tbsp tomato purée/paste

1.2l/40fl oz/5 cups chicken or vegetable stock

1 tbsp cumin seeds (optional)

sea salt and freshly ground black pepper

plain yogurt, to serve

Preheat the oven to 200°C/400°F/gas 6.

Place the carrots, onions and garlic cloves in a bowl and toss them in the olive oil along with some salt and pepper. Spread out in a roasting tray and roast on the top shelf of the oven for 10 minutes. Take the tray out and toss the vegetables to turn them, then return to the oven to cook for a further 15 minutes.

When cooked, tip the roasted vegetables into a large saucepan and add the tomatoes, red lentils and fresh dill. Place the pan over a medium heat and stir in the tomato purée/paste, followed by the stock. Bring to the boil, then turn the heat down and simmer gently for 10–15 minutes. Meanwhile, to toast the cumin seeds, if using, simply cook them in a frying pan (no oil is needed) over a medium heat until they just begin to smoke and release a strong spicy aroma. Tip out of the pan and leave to one side.

Season the soup well with salt and pepper, then pour it into a blender or use a hand-held/immersion blender to blend to a thick, smooth consistency.

Serve in bowls or deep mugs with a drizzle of plain yogurt and a sprinkling of the toasted cumin seeds, if using.

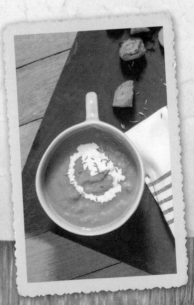

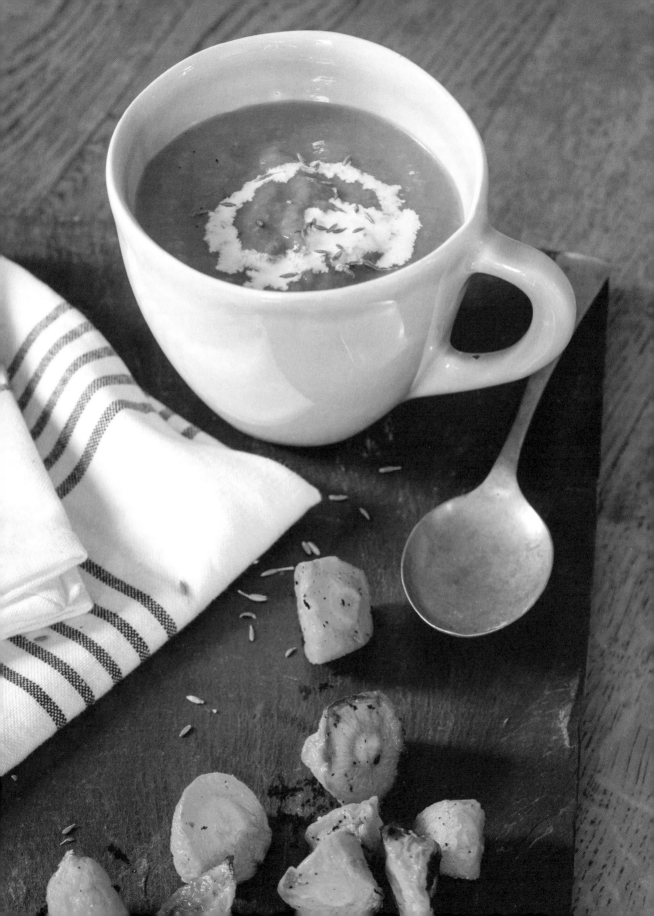

WILD GARLIC, LEEK AND PEA SOUP

READY IN **30** MINUTES

SERVES 4

55g/2oz/¼ cup butter

2 banana shallots, sliced

1 leek, sliced

850ml/30fl oz/3½ cups vegetable or chicken stock

480g/1lb 1oz/3½ cups peas or petit pois (fresh or frozen)

85g/3oz wild garlic leaves

12 basil leaves

1 Little Gem lettuce, shredded

squeeze of lemon juice

sea salt and freshly ground black pepper

Wild garlic, minerally and pungent, only has a short season, which coincides perfectly with the appearance of young summer vegetables. This recipe seizes the opportunity to make a wonderfully fresh and vibrant kitchen garden meal. Equally delicious cold or warm, serve this soup with a sprinkle of goats' cheese, toasted pine nuts or a drizzle of basil oil, depending on what you have.

Melt the butter in a large saucepan and, when sizzling, add the shallots. Cook for about 5 minutes until soft and translucent. Add the leek to the pan and stir to coat in the butter. Cook gently for 5–10 minutes, loosely covered with a lid, stirring every so often to stop the vegetables sticking to the bottom of the pan. Meanwhile, heat the stock until hot.

Tip in the peas, followed by the hot stock. Bring to the boil, turn the heat down, and then simmer gently for 5 minutes.

Carefully wash the wild garlic leaves, then shred them into ribbons along with the basil. Add to the pan, followed by the lettuce.

Season with salt and pepper and simmer for 2 minutes. Pour the soup into a blender or use a hand-held/immersion blender and blend until smooth. Pour it back into the pan to heat through again. Add the lemon juice and more salt and pepper if needed.

RED PEPPER, CHILLI AND TOMATO SOUP

The gentle sweetness of the peppers in this soup is complemented by the fiery chillies and rich tomatoes. Adding butter/lima beans gives a smooth, velvety consistency and means it's an altogether more filling meal.

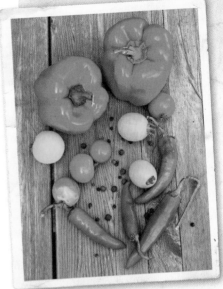

Heat a few glugs of rapeseed/canola oil in a large saucepan. Add the onion and garlic and cook over a medium heat for 2–3 minutes before adding the peppers and chillies. Cook for another 5 minutes, stirring every so often until the vegetables are softened.

Add the tomato purée/paste and thyme, and stir well. Add the tomatoes, followed by the butter/lima beans and a little salt and pepper. Place a lid on the pan and cook for 10 minutes.

Pour the stock into the pan, bring to the boil and return the lid to the pan. Simmer gently for 10 minutes. Take the pan off the heat and pour into a blender or use a hand-held/immersion blender to blend to a smooth purée. Add the sugar and vinegar and taste to check the seasoning, adding more salt and pepper if needed.

Serve in bowls topped with a drizzle of olive oil and some torn fresh basil or chilli/hot pepper flakes.

SERVES 4

READY IN **30** MINUTES

rapeseed/canola oil, for frying

1 onion, chopped

2 garlic cloves, chopped

2 red peppers, deseeded and chopped

2 red chillies, deseeded and chopped

2 tsp tomato purée/paste

1 tsp dried thyme

400g/14oz fresh tomatoes, roughly chopped

400g/14oz canned butter/lima beans, drained

750ml/26fl oz/3 cups vegetable stock

pinch of sugar

1 tbsp red wine vinegar

sea salt and freshly ground black pepper

olive oil, for drizzling

fresh basil or chilli/hot pepper flakes, for sprinkling

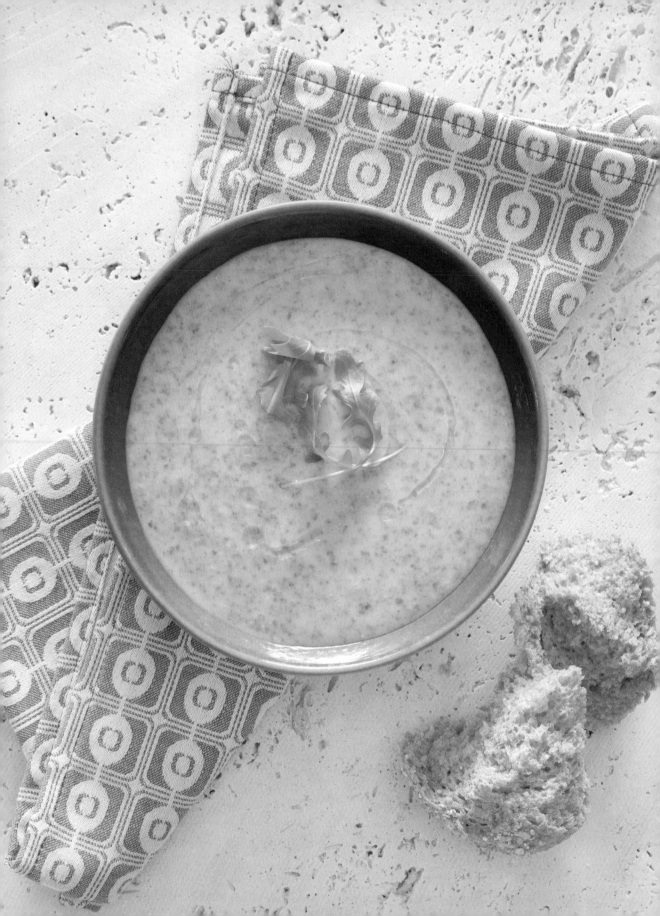

LITTLE GEM, CUCUMBER AND ROCKET SOUP

This couldn't be a more English soup, making the most of summery garden ingredients. It is unusual to cook lettuce and rocket/arugula, but the short cooking time allows them to keep their wonderful freshness. It's quite a light meal so for supper perhaps serve it with some warm focaccia, a crusty baguette or some home-made garlic bread.

Melt the butter in a saucepan and add the shallots. Cook gently for 5 minutes until the shallots have softened and turned translucent. Stir in the cucumber and potatoes and then pour in the stock. Bring to the boil, turn down the heat, and simmer, covered with a lid, for 10–12 minutes until the potato is soft enough to break easily if pressed with the back of a fork.

Tip in the lettuce, rocket/arugula, parsley and mint. Season with salt and pepper and stir well. Bring back to the boil, turn down the heat, and simmer gently for 2 minutes.

Tip the soup into a blender and purée until smooth. Do this in batches if you need to, returning the soup to the pan once puréed. Stir in the crème fraîche and taste to check the seasoning, adding more salt or pepper if needed.

Return the pan to the heat and bring almost to a simmer, being careful not to let it boil.

Serve with a drizzle of olive oil and a few extra rocket/arugula leaves scattered over and with warm bread.

SERVES 4

55g/2oz/¼ cup butter

2 banana shallots, chopped

½ large cucumber, deseeded and chopped

3 white potatoes (about 300g/10½oz), peeled and chopped

750ml/26fl oz/3 cups vegetable stock

2 Little Gem lettuces, shredded

115g/4oz/3 cups rocket/arugula, plus extra to serve

1 tbsp chopped parsley leaves

12 mint leaves, finely sliced

2 tbsp crème fraîche

sea salt and freshly ground black pepper

olive oil, for drizzling

crusty bread, to serve

NOTE: This soup is also delicious cold. Follow the same method above, but leave the soup to cool once you've stirred in the crème fraîche. Chill in the fridge until ready to serve.

ASPARAGUS, BROCCOLI AND PROSCIUTTO SALAD WITH CAPER AND HERB DRESSING

Seasonal asparagus should really remain as unadulterated as possible. In this salad, garden herbs, good-quality olive oil and a slice of earthy ham bring the asparagus to life without overpowering its delicate flavour. Dressing the vegetables while still warm intensifies the flavour of the dressing, too.

SERVES 4

4 eggs

300g/10½oz asparagus spears

300g/10½oz Tenderstem broccoli/broccolini

8 slices of prosciutto

handful of pine nuts, to serve

FOR THE DRESSING

handful of parsley

handful of tarragon

2 tbsp capers

1 tsp Dijon mustard

3 tbsp extra virgin olive oil, plus extra to serve

1 tbsp lemon juice, plus extra to serve

sea salt and freshly ground black pepper

Bring to the boil two pans of water – a small one for the eggs and a larger one for the vegetables.

When the smaller pan of water is simmering, gently drop in the eggs and cook for 6½ minutes. Remove from the pan and set aside.

Meanwhile, snap or cut the woody ends from the asparagus and discard. Blanch the asparagus and broccoli/broccolini in the boiling water until only just cooked – you still want the spears to have a bit of bite. This should take not much longer than 3–4 minutes.

While the vegetables are cooking, place the parsley, tarragon and capers on a board and chop together until quite fine. In a small bowl combine the chopped herb mixture with the mustard, olive oil, lemon juice and a little salt and pepper, stirring well.

Drain the vegetables into a large bowl, and while still warm, toss the herb and caper dressing through.

Peel the shell from the boiled eggs and cut them into quarters. Pile the asparagus, broccoli, prosciutto and eggs onto plates in layers. Scatter over a few pine nuts, drizzle over a little more olive oil or lemon juice, and add a sprinkling of salt and pepper.

NOTE: Crispy proscuitto is also great with this salad. Grill/broil slices for a minute or two laid flat on a baking sheet or place in a hot frying pan until they turn crispy and crunchy. Place on top of the salad.

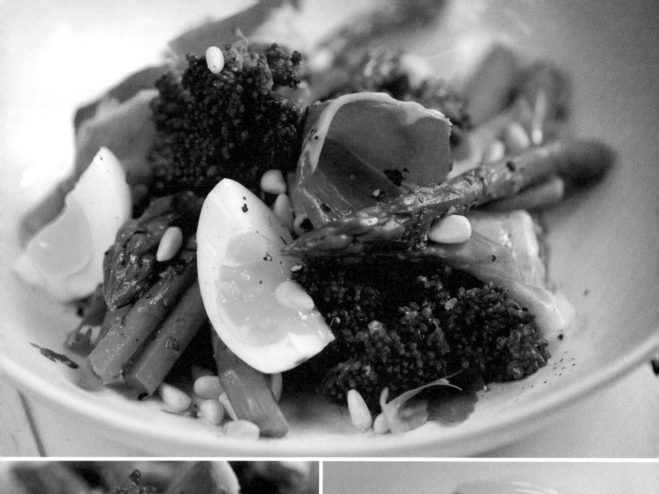
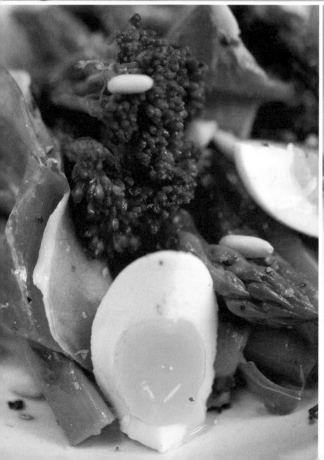
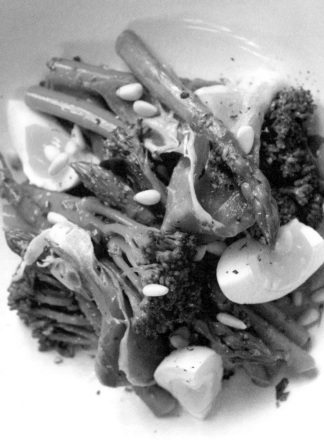

STRAWBERRY, FENNEL AND SMOKED CHICKEN SALAD

This recipe was created for Wimbledon week, which coincides with the British strawberry season hitting its peak. The summery flavours are perfect for a warm sunny evening, the heady sweet strawberries balanced by fresh fennel and bitter radicchio or red chicory leaves.

SERVES 4

50g/1¾oz/¾ cup flaked/sliced almonds

2 small fennel bulbs (about 400g/14oz)

150g/5½oz/1½ cups strawberries

handful of mint leaves

2 radicchio/red chicory lettuces

handful of rocket/arugula leaves

300g/10½oz smoked chicken

Pecorino or Parmesan cheese, to serve

FOR THE DRESSING

1 tbsp balsamic vinegar

3 tbsp extra virgin olive oil

pinch of caster/superfine sugar

zest of ½ lemon

sea salt and freshly ground black pepper

READY IN 15 MINUTES

Preheat the oven to 180°C/350°F/gas 4.

Scatter the flaked/sliced almonds on a baking sheet and bake for 5–6 minutes until golden.

Cut the fennel bulbs in half, remove the cores, and slice the leaves finely. Reserve any feathery tops to add to the salad later.

Wash, hull and slice the strawberries and shred the mint leaves into fine ribbons.

Make the dressing by whisking together the balsamic vinegar and olive oil with the sugar, lemon zest and a grinding of salt and pepper. Leave to one side.

Roughly tear the radicchio/red chicory into a bowl and add the rocket/arugula leaves. Tear the smoked chicken into small strips and add to the bowl along with the fennel, strawberries and mint.

Drizzle over the dressing and toss everything together thoroughly, adding any fennel tops you had kept back earlier.

Serve with the flaked/sliced almonds scattered over the top and a few shavings of Pecorino or Parmesan cheese.

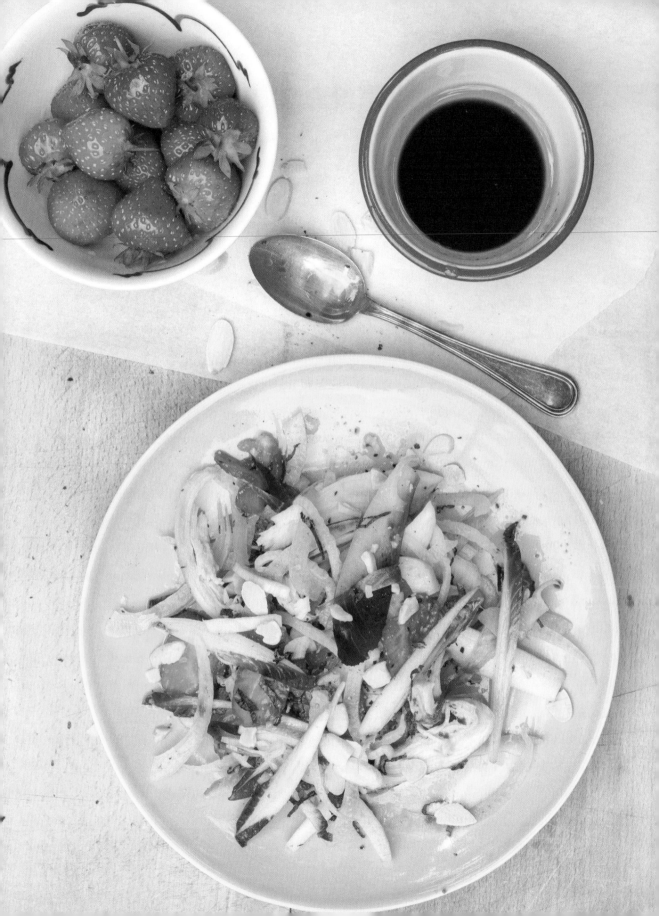

CHICKEN, BUTTERNUT SQUASH AND CHIVE SALAD

SERVES 4

1 butternut squash, peeled, deseeded, and chopped into 2cm/1in chunks

rapeseed/canola oil, for cooking

55g/2oz/½ cup walnut halves

450g/1lb cooked chicken or 4 chicken breasts

100g/3½oz/2 cups spinach leaves

20 pitted black olives

bunch of chives, chopped into 2cm/¾in lengths

sea salt and freshly ground black pepper

FOR THE DRESSING

1 tsp Dijon mustard

1 tbsp red wine vinegar

½ tsp honey

3 tbsp olive oil

1 garlic clove, crushed

This is a great way to use up leftover roast chicken. If your fridge is bare though, it takes no time to chargrill some for this salad. I like the mild, mineral flavour of the spinach leaves against the squash and olives but really, you can use any combination of green leaves you like – rocket/arugula, watercress or chicory/Belgian endive, for instance.

Preheat the oven to 200°C/400°F/gas 6.

Toss the butternut squash in a little rapeseed/canola oil, salt and pepper and roast on a baking sheet for 30 minutes, or until tender.

Meanwhile, spread the walnuts on a second baking sheet and bake for 8–10 minutes until golden. Remove from the oven and leave to one side. If you are cooking fresh chicken, rub a little oil, salt and pepper into each breast. Heat a griddle/grill pan and cook for 4–5 minutes on each side or until cooked through. Leave to one side.

To make the dressing, whisk together the mustard, vinegar, honey, olive oil and garlic and season with salt and pepper.

Shred the cooked chicken and place in a large serving bowl with the spinach, olives, chives and walnuts. When the butternut squash is cooked, add it to the bowl straight from the oven. Drizzle over the dressing, toss everything together well and pile onto plates.

NOTE: If you have some goats' cheese in the fridge, then this is delicious with a little crumbled over the top.

DUCK, GRAPEFRUIT AND SESAME SALAD

Bittersweet grapefruit goes perfectly with rich duck in this warm, winter leaf salad. Duck breasts are usually quite large, with one easily serving two people, so in this recipe there are only two duck breasts between four. You could also add warm potatoes to the salad to make it a more substantial meal.

Preheat the oven to 200°C/400°F/gas 6.

Using a sharp knife, score the skin of each duck breast and season on both sides. Place in a cold frying pan, skin-side down over a medium heat. Cook until the skin becomes crispy, pouring away any excess fat as you go, and then flip the duck breasts over, cooking for another minute or two to seal the underside. Place on a baking sheet and roast for 8–10 minutes until cooked (the duck should still be pink in the middle). Leave to rest for 5–10 minutes, covered with foil.

While the duck is cooking, tip the sesame seeds into a small pan and toast over a medium heat for 1–2 minutes until they turn a deep golden colour.

Make the dressing by placing the garlic, ginger, honey, sherry vinegar, soy sauce and olive oil in a small bowl and whisking together well, adding salt and pepper to taste.

Carefully peel the grapefruits and cut into segments, cutting away and discarding any white pith.

Roughly tear the chicory/Belgian endive into a large bowl along with the spinach or beet leaves and watercress.

Slice the duck and add to the salad along with the shallot, grapefruit and most of the toasted sesame seeds. Pour over the dressing, gently toss everything together and serve with the remaining sesame seeds scattered on top.

SERVES 4

2 large duck breasts
(or 3–4 small ones)

2 tbsp sesame seeds

2 red or white grapefruits

2 heads of chicory/Belgian endive

2 large handfuls of baby spinach
or beet leaves

handful of watercress

1 large shallot, very finely sliced

sea salt and freshly ground
black pepper

FOR THE DRESSING

1 garlic clove, grated

2cm/¾in piece of root ginger,
peeled and grated

1 tsp honey

1 tbsp sherry vinegar

1 tbsp tamari soy sauce

3 tbsp olive oil

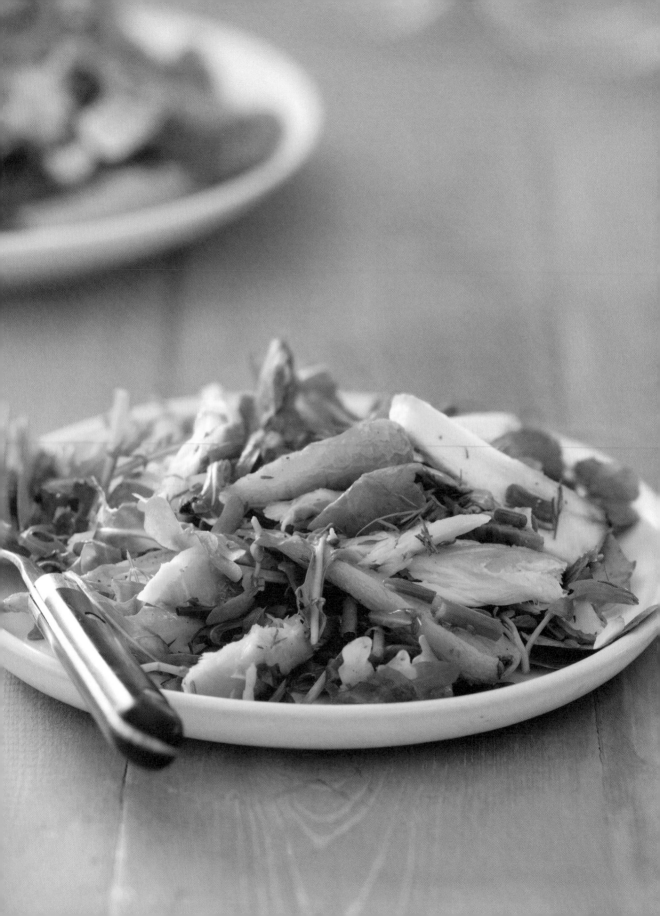

WARM MACKEREL AND ROASTED ROOT VEGETABLE SALAD

The warm roasted carrots and parsnips lightly wilt the leaves as this salad is tossed together, and the heat brings out the fresh, herby flavours in the dressing. Don't bother to peel the vegetables; the cooked skin has a lovely chewy texture. The dill and chives add depth but you can use any mixture of herbs you have.

Preheat the oven to 190°C/375°F/gas 5.

Slice the carrots in half lengthways and cut the parsnips into wedges so that the pieces are roughly the same size as the carrots. Toss in a little rapeseed/canola oil with the cumin seeds and add salt and pepper. Spread out in a roasting tray and roast at the top of the oven for 25 minutes until cooked through and slightly caramelized at the edges.

Meanwhile, make the dressing. Combine the lemon juice and mustard in a small bowl with a little salt and pepper. Whisk in the rapeseed/canola oil.

Place the chives, dill, rocket/arugula, watercress and capers in a large salad bowl. Remove the skin from the mackerel fillets and break the flesh into bite-size pieces with your fingers, adding to the salad bowl as you go.

When the carrots and parsnips are cooked, tip them straight into the salad. Pour over the dressing and toss everything together well.

READY IN **30** MINUTES

SERVES 4

450g/1lb baby carrots

3 parsnips

rapeseed/canola oil, for cooking

3 tsp cumin seeds

handful of chives, roughly chopped

handful of dill, roughly chopped

100g/3½oz/2 cups rocket/arugula

100g/3½oz/2 cups watercress

2 tbsp capers, roughly chopped

4 smoked mackerel fillets

sea salt and freshly ground black pepper

FOR THE DRESSING

juice of ½ lemon

1 heaped tsp Dijon mustard

3 tbsp rapeseed/canola oil

WARM SALMON, WATERCRESS AND GREEN BEAN SALAD

A quick and versatile supper that you can easily adapt by adding your favourite ingredients: a soft-boiled egg, roast baby beetroot/beet, black olives, rocket/arugula or lambs' lettuce would all work well. Or try replacing the salmon with freshly grilled mackerel or tuna.

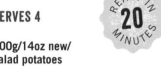

SERVES 4

400g/14oz new/
salad potatoes

4 salmon fillets

olive oil, for drizzling

200g/7oz green beans

115g/4oz/2 cups watercress

small handful of chives, chopped

2 tbsp chopped parsley

sea salt and freshly ground
black pepper

FOR THE DRESSING

½ garlic clove, crushed

1 tsp Dijon mustard

1 tsp honey

1 tbsp lemon juice and a little
grated zest

3 tbsp olive oil

Preheat the oven to 190°C/375°F/gas 5.

Place the potatoes in a saucepan, cover with water, bring to the boil and cook for 12–15 minutes until tender. Drain and return to the pan.

Meanwhile, place the salmon fillets on a foil-lined baking sheet, drizzle over a little olive oil and season with salt and pepper. Roast in the middle of the oven for 12–15 minutes until just cooked through.

While the potatoes and salmon are cooking make the salad dressing. Mix the garlic, mustard and honey and a little salt and pepper in a small bowl. Using a fork, whisk in the lemon juice and zest and lastly the olive oil. Taste and add more salt and pepper, if needed.

Bring a second pan of salted water to the boil and cook the beans for 1–2 minutes until just tender. Drain the beans and add them to same pan as the potatoes. Pour the dressing over the beans and potatoes while they are still warm, then put on the lid and gently shake the pan to distribute the dressing evenly.

Tip the potatoes and beans into a large salad bowl, add the watercress, chives and parsley and toss together. Flake the cooked salmon onto the salad, gently mix together and serve sprinkled with a little salt and pepper.

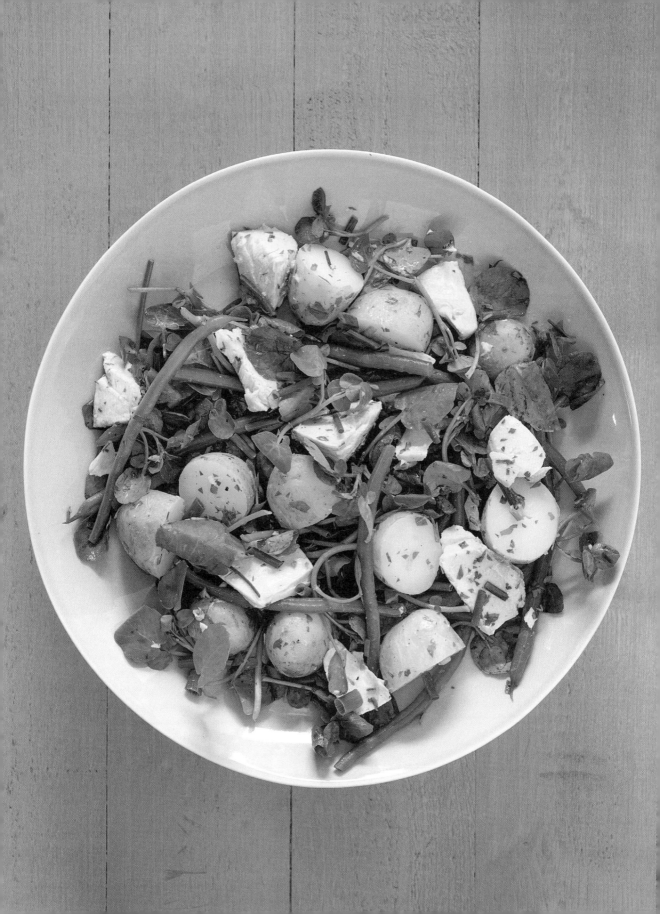

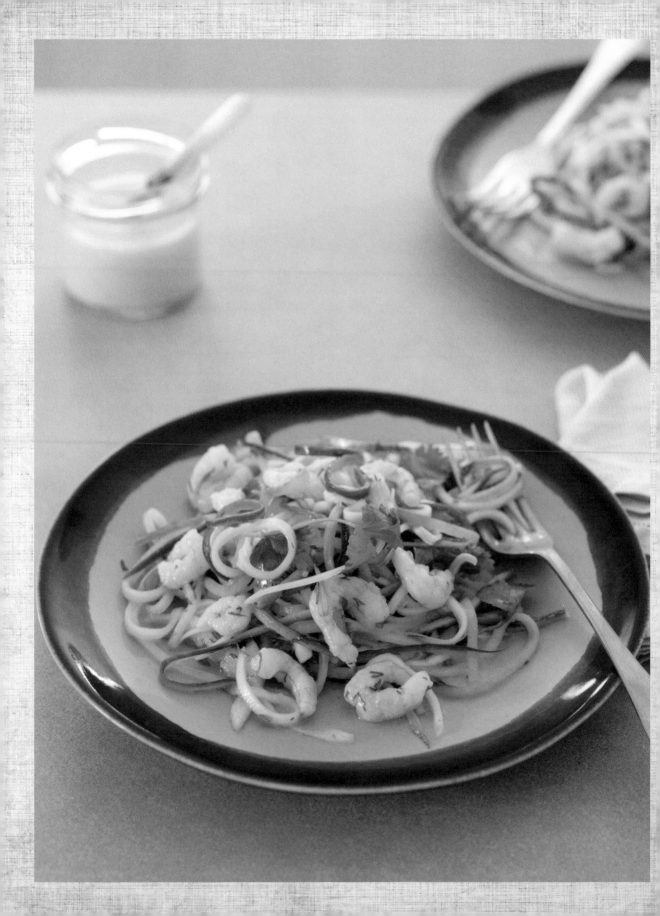

PRAWN, COURGETTE AND CORIANDER SALAD

This is a beautiful salad, laced with whole coriander/cilantro leaves and long strips of courgette/zucchini and cucumber. It is very quick to make, especially if you use a spiralizer or julienne peeler. For anyone fond of a bit of heat, do add the finely chopped green chilli.

READY IN 15 MINUTES

Begin by shredding the courgette/zucchini and cucumber lengthways into fine strips using a spiralizer or julienne peeler. Discard the seeds when you reach them. Place the strips in a large bowl with the shallot, chilli (if using), dill, coriander/cilantro leaves and prawns/shrimp.

To make the dressing, whisk together the rapeseed/canola oil, yogurt, lemon juice and fish sauce. Drizzle this over the salad and toss everything together well. I find this easiest to do with tongs or a pair of forks so that everything becomes evenly coated in dressing.

Pile onto serving plates and top with a little more coriander/cilantro.

SERVES 4

3 large courgettes/zucchini

1 large cucumber

1 banana shallot, very finely sliced

1 green chilli, deseeded and finely chopped (optional)

4 sprigs of dill, leaves only, chopped

2 handfuls of coriander/cilantro leaves, plus extra for sprinkling

400g/14oz small cooked peeled prawns/shrimp

FOR THE DRESSING

55ml/2fl oz/¼ cup rapeseed/canola oil

2 tbsp plain yogurt

squeeze of lemon juice

2 tbsp fish sauce

CRAB, AVOCADO AND RADISH SALAD

SERVES 4

500g/1lb 2oz/4½ cups
fresh white crab meat

juice of ½ lemon

2 ripe avocados

2 Little Gem lettuces

100g/3½oz/3 cups rocket/
arugula leaves

bunch of radishes, washed
and quartered

sea salt and freshly ground
black pepper

FOR THE DRESSING

1 egg yolk

½ tsp Dijon mustard

150ml/5fl oz/⅔ cup rapeseed/canola
or vegetable oil

2 tbsp plain yogurt

handful of tarragon, chopped

handful of chives, chopped

NOTE: If aniseedy tarragon
isn't your favourite flavour
then only use chives or replace
with a little parsley or chervil.

Fresh, bright and herby, this salad may sound rather light but is surprisingly filling. Served with a bowl of new, salad potatoes or a softly poached egg it becomes quite substantial, and on a warm evening you won't need much more than a glass of white wine and slice of crusty bread alongside.

Tip the crab meat into a bowl and season with salt and pepper and the lemon juice.

To make the dressing, drop the egg yolk into a small bowl and add the mustard and a grind of salt and pepper. Slowly pour in the oil while whisking with a fork. Stir in the yogurt and then about three-quarters of the chopped herbs. Taste and add an extra squeeze of lemon juice, if needed. Leave the dressing to one side.

Halve the avocados, remove the pits and scoop the flesh out of the skin into bite-size pieces using a teaspoon.

Rip the Little Gem lettuces into manageable pieces and pile onto a plate with the rocket/arugula leaves, followed by the avocados, crab and radishes. Drizzle over the dressing and scatter over the remaining tarragon and chives.

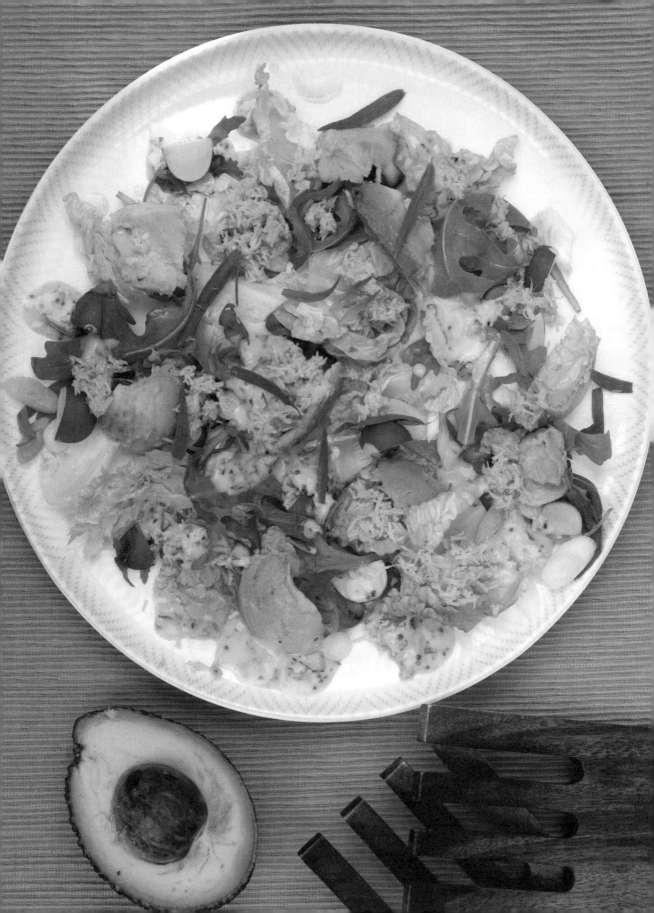

TWO-BEAN, GOATS' CHEESE, CHERRY AND HAZELNUT SALAD

SERVES 4

2 tbsp hazelnuts
(unpeeled or peeled)

200g/7oz runner beans or
sugar snap peas/snow peas

200g/7oz fine/French beans

1–2 goats' cheeses, cut into
8 slices, each 2cm/¾in thick

2 radicchio/red chicory lettuces

handful of chives, chopped

85g/3oz/⅓ cup cherries,
pitted and halved

FOR THE DRESSING

juice and zest ½ lemon

3 tbsp hazelnut oil

1 tsp wholegrain mustard

pinch of brown sugar

sea salt and freshly ground
black pepper

NOTE: This recipe works
very well with cooked chicken
in place of the goats' cheese.
Simply add 400g/14oz
of shredded chicken to the
salad leaves when you toss
everything together.

Green beans and cherries combine well with hazelnuts in this warm, autumnal salad. A squeeze of lemon juice and a few chives give a fresh sharpness against the earthy hazelnuts. If hazelnut oil proves elusive then alternatives such as walnut, rapeseed/canola or olive will work well. Make sure you buy goats' cheese with rind that can be sliced into fat discs rather than a soft cream cheese type.

Preheat the oven to 190°C/375°F/gas 5.

Spread out the hazelnuts on a baking sheet and roast for 5 minutes until golden. Remove from the oven, chop roughly and leave to one side.

Remove the tops and tails of the beans; if the runner beans are large or old you may also need to run a knife along their long edge to remove the tough stringy part. Slice the runner beans diagonally into long strips and leave the fine/French beans and sugar snap/snow peas (if using) whole.

Bring a pan of salted water to the boil and add the beans. Cook for 3–4 minutes until just tender. Drain and cool under cold running water.

To make the dressing, whisk together the lemon juice, hazelnut oil and mustard along with the sugar and a little salt and pepper. Taste and add more salt and pepper if needed.

Preheat the grill/broiler to its highest setting. Lay the slices of goats' cheese on a foil-lined sheet and place under the grill/broiler for 3 minutes until the cheese has softened and turned golden. Leave to one side.

Roughly tear the radicchio/chicory leaves into a large bowl and add the beans and chives. Pour over the dressing, toss to mix well and pile onto plates. Carefully place the goats' cheese on top. Scatter over the hazelnuts and cherries and finish with the lemon zest.

QUINOA, AVOCADO AND SPINACH SALAD

Full of contrasting textures, this feels to me about as healthy as a salad can get, with delicious roasted seeds, chunks of creamy avocado and nutty grains of quinoa. The trick is to dress the quinoa while still warm, which slightly wilts the spinach leaves and really allows the flavours in the salad to come through.

Preheat the oven to 200°C/400°F/gas 6.

Scatter the pumpkin seeds on a baking sheet and roast for 8–10 minutes until golden. Leave to one side.

Meanwhile, in a small saucepan, pour 400ml/14 fl oz/1¾ cups boiling water over the quinoa. Bring to the boil, turn the heat down, and then simmer gently, covered with a lid, for 10–12 minutes until the water has been absorbed and the quinoa is cooked. Drain, then tip into a large bowl while you prepare the rest of the ingredients.

To make the dressing, combine the chilli, garlic, lemon juice and olive oil in a small bowl and whisk together, adding a little salt. Pour this over the quinoa and stir in the cranberries, followed by the spinach, avocado, basil and roasted pumpkin seeds. Mix well and taste to check if the salad needs more salt or pepper.

Either serve straight away, while still slightly warm, or leave to cool.

READY IN 20 MINUTES

SERVES 4

55g/2oz/¼ cup pumpkin seeds

225g/8oz/1⅓ cups quinoa

55g/2oz/¼ cup dried cranberries

55g/2oz/1 cup spinach leaves

1 large avocado, peeled, pitted and diced

12 basil leaves, sliced

FOR THE DRESSING

1 red chilli, finely chopped

2 garlic cloves, crushed

2 tbsp lemon juice

4 tbsp olive oil

sea salt and freshly ground black pepper

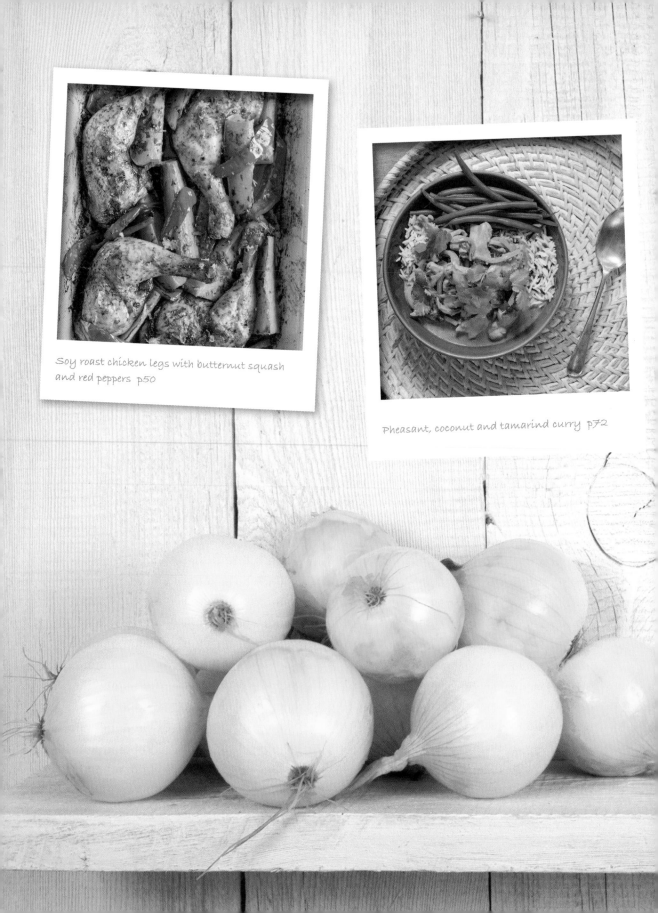

Soy roast chicken legs with butternut squash
and red peppers p50

Pheasant, coconut and tamarind curry p72

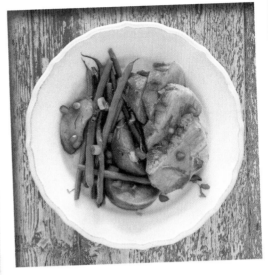

Duck breasts with peaches and balsamic vinegar p71

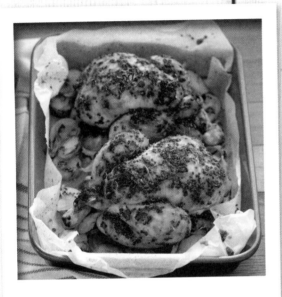

Honey and mustard-glazed poussin p67

POULTRY

SOY ROAST CHICKEN LEGS WITH BUTTERNUT SQUASH AND RED PEPPERS

This is one of my favourite after-work meals. Colourful and full of flavour, it takes hardly any time to prepare and is made up of ingredients you might already have in the fridge or cupboard.

Imagine one of those combinations that hits all of your taste buds at once; the sticky garlic and soy marinade caramelizes on the outer edges of the chicken and butternut squash while the peppers, oregano and lemon bring everything sharply to life.

Serve it straight from the oven with a crunchy green salad and, if you're really hungry, some mashed potato.

SERVES 4

READY IN 40 MINUTES

1 small butternut squash, chopped into wedges (there is no need to peel)

4 chicken legs

1 red pepper, sliced

4 tbsp soy sauce

2 tbsp olive oil

2 garlic cloves, crushed

2 tsp dried oregano

pinch of brown sugar

zest of 1 lemon

small handful of parsley, chopped

freshly ground black pepper

Preheat the oven to 200°C/400°F/gas 6.

Spread out the butternut squash wedges, chicken legs and red pepper in a deep roasting tray.

Mix together the soy sauce, olive oil, garlic, oregano and sugar in a small bowl and pour over the butternut squash, chicken and red pepper, turning everything over to coat all sides in the mixture. Season with plenty of black pepper, then turn the chicken legs skin-side up.

Place in the middle of the oven and cook for 30 minutes or until the squash is soft and the chicken skin brown and crispy. Take the tray out of the oven and scatter with the lemon zest and chopped parsley.

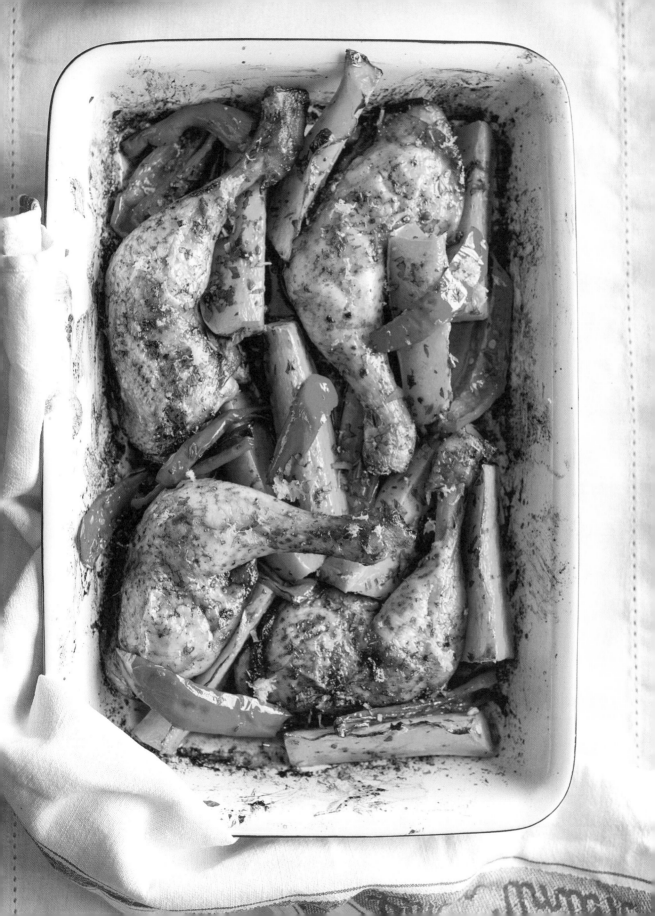

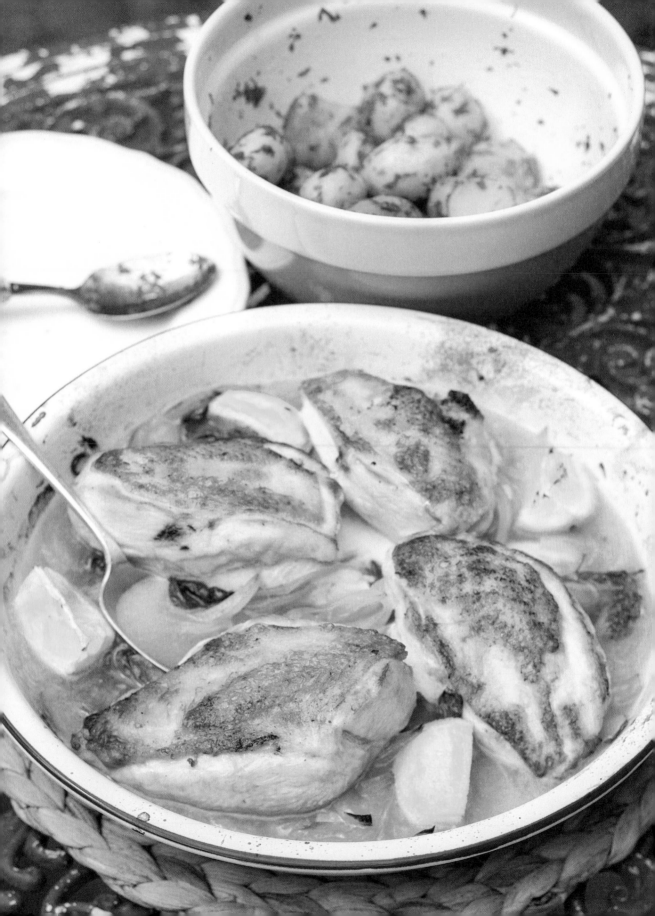

CHICKEN WITH RICOTTA, LEMON AND BASIL

A vibrant, summery weeknight recipe that is delicious served with steaming new/salad potatoes. Although I particularly love the mild flavour of ricotta, you can substitute other soft cheeses such as mascarpone or goats' cheese.

Preheat the oven to 200°C/400°F/gas 6.

Finely slice half of the basil leaves, leaving the other half on their stems for later. In a small bowl mix the ricotta cheese with the basil, the zest of 1 lemon and a little salt and pepper.

Use a sharp knife to cut a horizontal pocket into each chicken breast, being careful not to cut all the way through. Stuff a little of the ricotta mixture into the pockets with a teaspoon, being careful not to overfill.

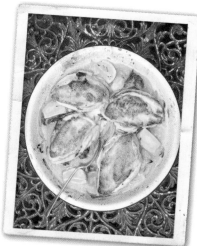

Heat a little oil in a large frying pan and add the chicken breasts, skin-side down. Fry for 2–3 minutes until the skin is golden and crisp. Flip onto the other side and cook for a further minute to lightly seal and then remove to a plate.

Return the pan to the heat and add the onion and garlic. Cook for about 5 minutes until well softened. Pour in the white wine and stock, add the bay leaves and bring to the boil. Simmer for a few minutes to reduce the liquid to a syrupy consistency. Add the double/heavy cream, stir well and season with salt and pepper.

Pour the contents of the pan into a casserole dish and place the chicken breasts on top, pushing them down into the sauce, skin-side up. Cut the remaining lemon into wedges and nestle them around the chicken along with the remaining basil.

Place on the middle shelf of the oven and cook for 15–20 minutes until the chicken is cooked through and the skins are nicely brown and crisp. Test if cooked by cutting into one of the breasts with a sharp knife to make sure the juices run clear.

NOTE: If you are avoiding cow's milk then use soft goats' or sheeps' cheese for the stuffing and simply omit the double/heavy cream from the recipe.

READY IN 40 MINUTES

SERVES 4

small bunch of basil

100g/3½oz/½ cup ricotta cheese

4 chicken breasts (skin on)

2 lemons

rapeseed/canola oil, for cooking

1 onion, sliced

1 garlic clove, crushed

170ml/5½fl oz/⅔ cup white wine

125ml/4fl oz/½ cup chicken stock

2 bay leaves

1 tbsp double/heavy cream

sea salt and freshly ground black pepper

ONE-POT CHICKEN WITH BACON, LEEKS AND PEAS

This one-pot chicken dish is full of the flavours of spring and takes only 40 minutes to cook. Be generous with the herbs and feel free to add your favourite green vegetables: asparagus tips, sliced baby courgettes/zucchini or broad/fava beans could all be added along with the peas.

SERVES 4

READY IN **40** MINUTES

rapeseed/canola oil, for cooking

8 skinless chicken thighs

100g/3½oz smoked streaky bacon, sliced

2 leeks, finely sliced

300ml/10½fl oz/1¼ cups chicken stock

300g/10½oz/2¼ cups frozen peas

2 tsp Dijon mustard

1 Little Gem lettuce, halved and finely shredded

large handful of tarragon, chopped

large handful of parsley, chopped

sea salt and freshly ground black pepper

steamed wild or brown rice and crème fraîche, to serve

Heat a little oil in a large casserole dish or lidded pan. Season the chicken thighs with salt and pepper and cook on both sides for 3–4 minutes until browned. Do this in two batches, removing the chicken pieces and reserving in a separate dish until later.

Put the bacon in the pan and cook for 1–2 minutes until crispy. Next, add the leeks and turn the heat down slightly, stirring frequently until the leeks have wilted and softened but are still bright green.

In a separate pan, heat the chicken stock until warm. Place the chicken pieces back into the pan with the leeks and pour over the warm stock. Stir well, bring to a gentle simmer, add the lid, and leave to bubble away for 10 minutes, stirring halfway through. Add the frozen peas, stir well, replace the lid and simmer gently for another 5 minutes until the chicken is cooked through.

Add the Dijon mustard, lettuce, tarragon and parsley and add plenty of black pepper. Stir well, bring back to a simmer, turn off the heat and replace the lid. Leave to stand for a minute or two before tasting to check the seasoning.

I serve this in deep bowls with steamed wild or brown rice and a dollop of crème fraîche on top.

NOTE: Chicken thighs (bone in or out) are best for this recipe as they have so much flavour, but you can use four chicken breasts, cut in half if you prefer, or even a whole, jointed chicken. Pheasant or guinea fowl would also work well but be careful not to cook for too long as the meat can dry out very quickly.

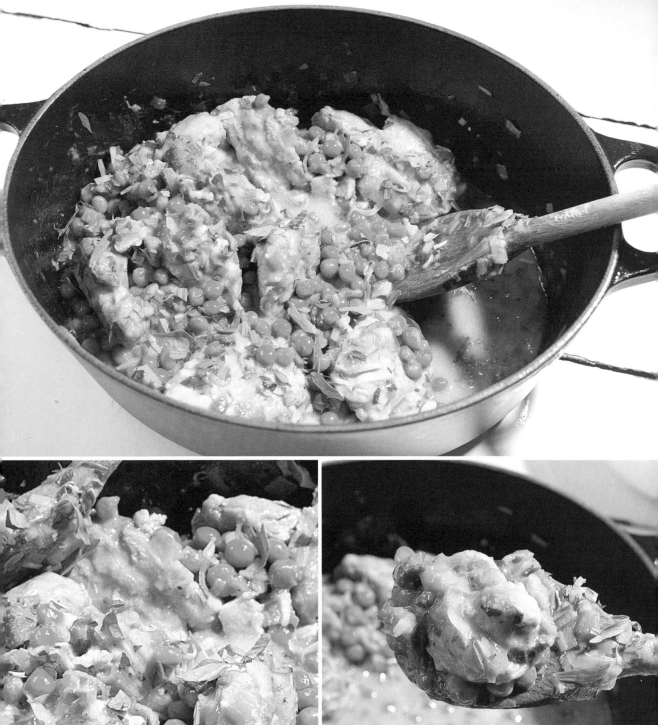
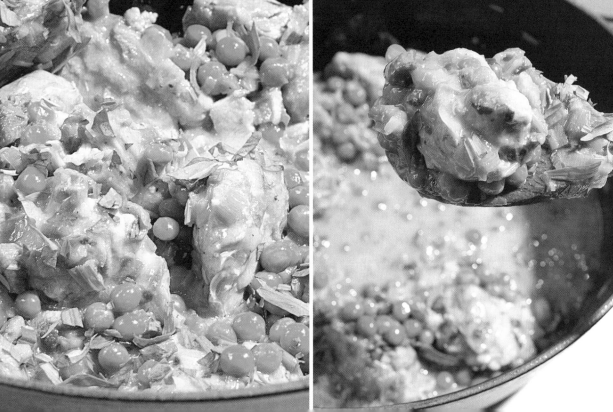

SICILIAN CHICKEN WITH FENNEL AND GREEN OLIVES

SERVES 4

rapeseed/canola oil, for cooking

8 skinless chicken thighs

50g/1¾oz bacon lardons or streaky bacon, diced

1 fennel bulb (about 200g/7oz), cored and finely sliced

1 onion, sliced

1 garlic clove, sliced

1 tsp tomato purée/paste

1 tsp dried oregano

800g/1lb 12oz/3½ cups canned chopped tomatoes

3 tbsp pitted green olives

1 tbsp capers (optional)

pinch of caster/granulated sugar

sea salt and freshly ground black pepper

handful of parsley, roughly chopped, for sprinkling

A one-pot supper made from store-cupboard ingredients, this is a hassle-free meal, delicious with couscous, rice or steamed potatoes and a bowl of green beans. If you can't find green olives then purple or black ones can replace them, and if you have a salty palate then a tablespoon of capers wouldn't go amiss.

Heat a little oil in a large casserole dish or lidded pan. Season the chicken thighs with salt and pepper and cook on both sides for 3–4 minutes until browned. Do this in two batches, removing the chicken pieces and reserving in a separate dish until later.

Put the bacon in the pan and cook for 1–2 minutes until crispy. Add the fennel, onion and garlic and cook for 5 minutes until the vegetables are softened and slightly coloured.

Stir in the tomato purée/paste and oregano, followed by the tomatoes, green olives, capers (if using) and sugar. Return the chicken to the pan. Add about 150ml/5fl oz/⅔ cup water to loosen the sauce if needed, and season well with salt and pepper. Add a lid, bring to the boil and simmer for 20 minutes until the chicken is cooked through.

Taste, adjust the seasoning if needed, and serve with the parsley scattered on top.

RED LENTIL AND CHICKEN SAAG

Spinach curries are one of my absolute favourites, especially combined with gently cooked lentils and, as in this recipe, fenugreek. Often, cream or yogurt is added to this sort of curry but there isn't any need unless you'd like that extra richness. I would serve this with wild basmati rice and mango chutney.

Heat the oil in a heavy based frying pan. Add the onion and cook for 2–3 minutes before adding the garlic and chilli; cook for another 5 minutes until softened. Stir in the tomato purée/paste, garam masala, turmeric and fenugreek, and after 1 minute, add the red lentils, stirring to coat them in spices and oil.

Add the chicken to the pan, stirring well over the heat for a few minutes to seal. Pour in the tomatoes, followed by the stock and some salt and pepper.

Bring to the boil, then turn down the heat to a gentle simmer. Tip in the spinach, stirring gently until they wilt into the sauce. Simmer gently for 20 minutes until the chicken and lentils are cooked through.

If the curry looks dry during cooking, add a little more stock. Adjust the seasoning to your taste and add double/heavy cream or yogurt if you like.

SERVES 4

2 tbsp rapeseed/canola oil

1 onion, finely chopped

2 garlic cloves, crushed

1 red chilli, deseeded and finely chopped

1 tsp tomato purée/paste

2 tsp garam masala

1 tsp ground turmeric

1 tsp ground fenugreek

115g/4oz/½ cup dried red lentils

500g/1lb 2oz chicken breast fillets, diced

400g/14oz/1¾ cups canned chopped tomatoes

400ml/14oz/1⅔ cups chicken stock

200g/7oz/4 cups spinach leaves

sea salt and freshly ground black pepper

2 tbsp double/heavy cream or yogurt, to serve (optional)

YOGURT-MARINATED CHICKEN WITH COURGETTE SLAW

A great way to make use of a glut of courgettes/zucchini, this slaw is fresh and bright and a great barbecue side dish. The yogurt and lemon tenderize the chicken, making it incredibly succulent.

SERVES 4

READY IN **40** MINUTES

2 garlic cloves, crushed

175ml/6fl oz/¾ cup plain yogurt

2 tbsp olive oil

juice and zest of ½ lemon

handful of parsley, finely chopped

500g/1lb 2oz chicken breast fillets

sea salt and freshly ground black pepper

FOR THE SLAW

2 tsp nigella (black onion) seeds

2 tbsp olive oil

1 tbsp white wine vinegar

pinch of brown sugar

squeeze of lemon juice

2 large courgettes/zucchini, grated

1 cucumber, grated

55g/2oz/1½ cups rocket/arugula

handful of mint leaves, chopped

To make the marinade for the chicken, combine the garlic with the yogurt, olive oil, lemon juice and zest and parsley in a small bowl. Season with salt and pepper and mix well.

Pour the yogurt mixture over the chicken pieces, mix to coat evenly and leave to marinate for 20 minutes while you make the slaw.

In a small pan, lightly toast the nigella seeds over a medium heat for 2 minutes until you can smell their strong aroma. Tip out of the pan and leave to one side.

Make the dressing for the slaw by whisking the olive oil with the white wine vinegar, sugar and a squeeze of lemon juice. Combine the courgettes/zucchini, cucumber, rocket/arugula and mint leaves in a large salad bowl. Add the nigella seeds and dressing and toss.

Preheat the grill/broiler to its highest setting. Lay the marinated chicken pieces out on a foil-lined baking sheet and cook for 5 minutes. Turn the chicken over and cook for a further 5 minutes until cooked all the way through and slightly golden at the edges. Serve with the slaw.

NOTE: This chicken is great cooked on a griddle/grill pan if you have one, or threaded onto a skewer and cooked on a barbecue.

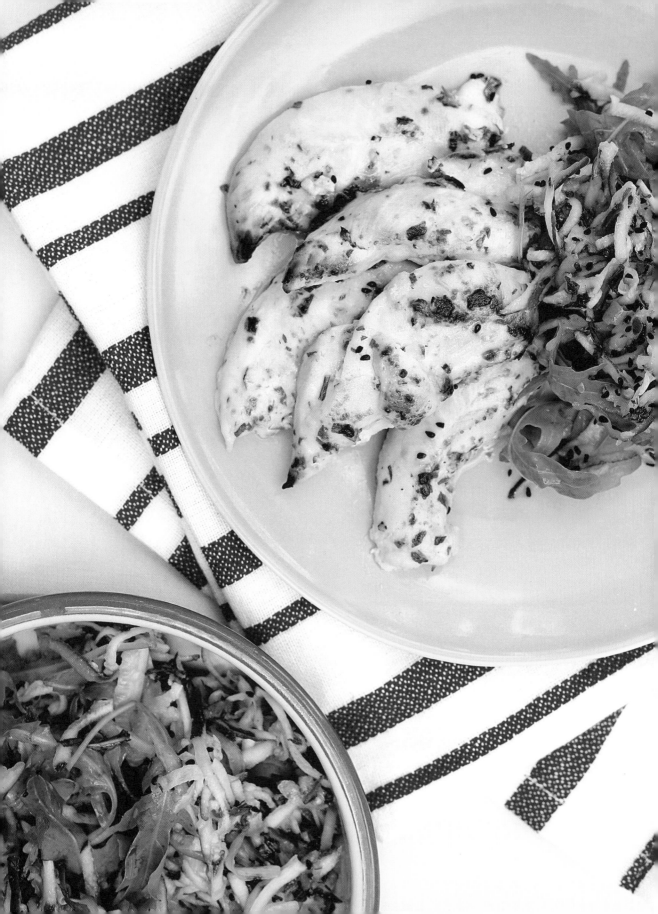

CHICKEN WITH MUSHROOMS AND TARRAGON

SERVES 4

rapeseed/canola oil, for cooking

4 chicken breasts (skin on)

1 large onion, finely sliced

4 large field mushrooms, sliced

225ml/8fl oz/scant 1 cup white wine

300ml/10½fl oz/1¼ cups double/
heavy cream

1 tsp Dijon mustard

handful of tarragon leaves,
roughly chopped

sea salt and freshly ground
black pepper

The bittersweet tarragon in this dish cuts through the cream to give a lovely piquancy to the sauce. The same sauce works very well with pheasant, guinea fowl or pork chops.

Heat 1 tablespoon of oil in a deep frying pan. Slice the chicken breasts in half diagonally, season with salt and pepper and fry skin-side down for 3–4 minutes until the skin is golden. Flip the chicken over and cook for a further minute on the flesh side. Remove from the pan and leave to one side.

Return the pan to the heat, add a little more oil, followed by the onion. Cook for 5 minutes until softened and slightly coloured. Add the mushrooms and cook for a further 5 minutes, stirring often and adding a little more oil if needed.

Pour in the white wine and simmer for 3–4 minutes until it turns slightly syrupy. Add the cream, mustard, most of the tarragon and some salt and pepper. Stir well, bring to a simmer and return the chicken pieces to the pan, skin-side up. Place a lid on the pan and cook gently for 10–12 minutes until the chicken is cooked through.

Serve with the remaining tarragon scattered over the top.

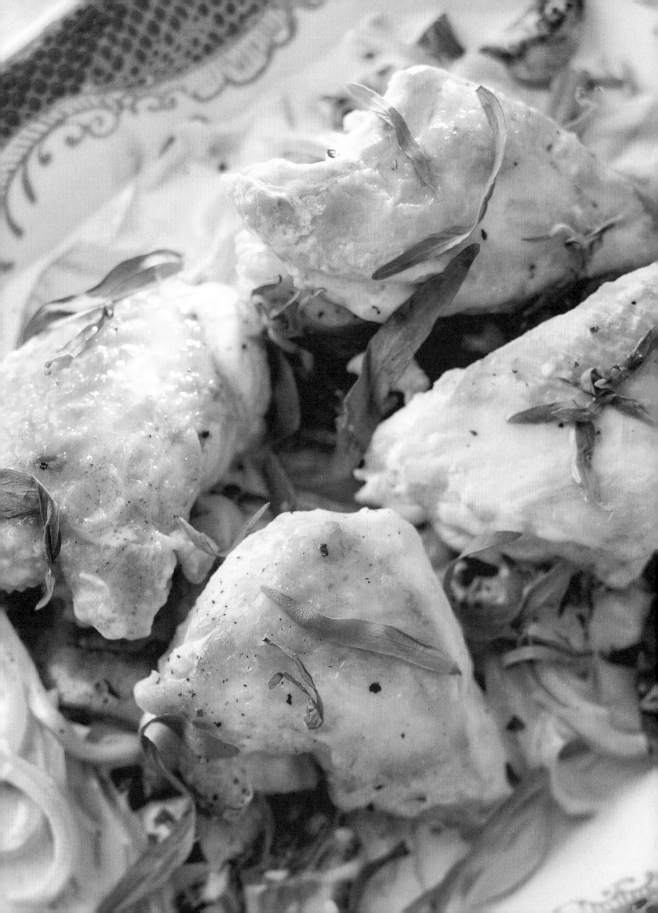

CHICKEN PUTTANESCA

Spicy, sweet and salty, this classic Italian sauce is full of taste bud-pleasing flavours that will liven up a pack of chicken thighs. Serve with spaghetti, rice or fluffy mashed potatoes and some green vegetables.

SERVES 4

READY IN **30** MINUTES

rapeseed/canola oil, for cooking

1 onion, finely chopped

1 garlic clove, chopped

1 red chilli, deseeded and finely chopped

8 chicken thigh fillets, halved

2 tsp tomato purée/paste

4 anchovies, chopped

400g/14oz/1¾ cups canned chopped tomatoes

1 tbsp capers

150ml/5fl oz/⅔ cup chicken or vegetable stock

2 tbsp pitted purple olives

brown sugar, to taste (optional)

freshly ground black pepper

handful of basil leaves, roughly torn, for sprinkling

Heat a little oil in a deep frying pan and add the onion. Cook for 5 minutes until softened, then add the garlic and chilli and cook for another 5 minutes.

Push the onion and garlic to the sides of the pan, turn up the heat a little and add the chicken pieces. Cook for 3–4 minutes, turning until the chicken colours a little and is sealed on all sides. Stir in the tomato purée/paste, followed by the anchovies, tomatoes, capers and stock and bring to the boil.

Place a lid loosely on top of the pan and simmer for 15 minutes, stirring occasionally, until the chicken is cooked through. Add the olives, some black pepper (the capers and anchovies mean you won't need to add salt) and taste to check the seasoning – add a pinch of sugar if there is any bitterness. Serve with the basil leaves scattered over.

NOTE: If you have leftover cooked chicken from a roast, then use this in place of the raw chicken thighs. Make the sauce as above and add the cooked chicken in the final few minutes.

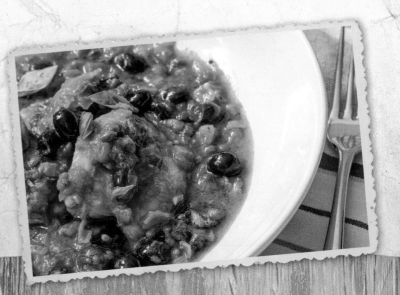

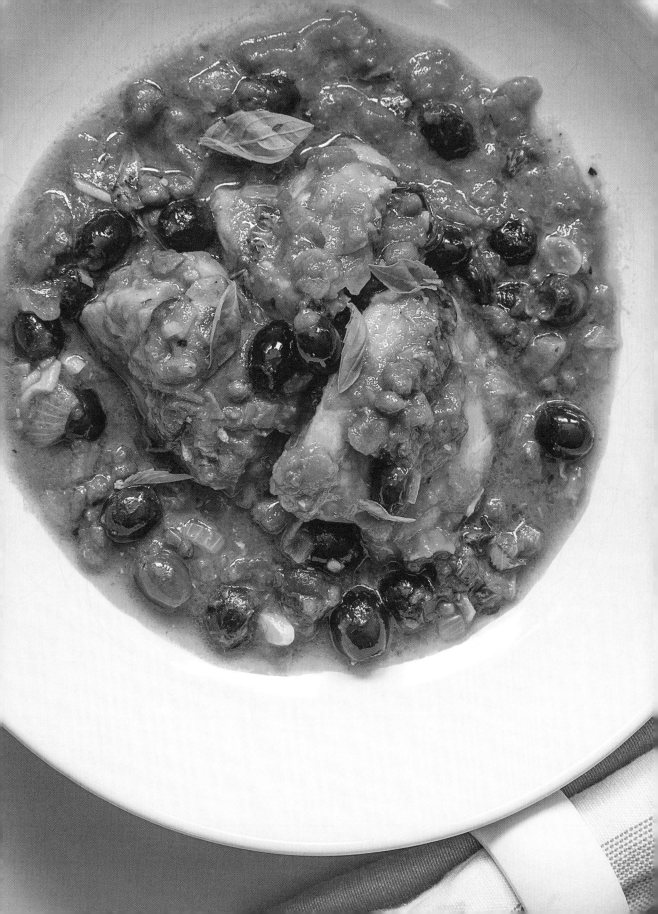

CHICKEN CIABATTA WITH HERBY TAHINI SLAW

READY IN **15** MINUTES

4 chicken breasts

1 tbsp olive oil, plus extra for rubbing

zest of ½ lemon

1 tsp oregano

1 tsp chilli powder

rapeseed/canola oil, for cooking

4 ciabatta rolls

sea salt and freshly ground black pepper

salad leaves, to serve

FOR THE SLAW

1 tbsp tahini

4 tbsp plain yogurt

juice of ½ lemon

1 tbsp olive oil

1 garlic clove, crushed

¼ red cabbage, finely shredded

¼ white cabbage, finely shredded

1 red onion, finely sliced

1 tbsp chopped parsley

1 tbsp chopped coriander/cilantro leaves

As sandwiches go this is a pretty healthy one, as it is packed full of vegetables. Made with yogurt and tahini, the slaw's dressing has a delicious nutty flavour without the richness of traditional coleslaw. Combined with salad leaves, lean chicken and raw cabbage it is nutritious as well as satisfying.

Lay the chicken breasts flat on a board and, using a sharp knife, slice each one horizontally in half to leave you with 8 slim escalopes. Place in a bowl with the olive oil, lemon zest, oregano, chilli powder and some salt and pepper. Rub the mixture into the chicken escalopes and leave to one side.

Make the dressing for the slaw by combining the tahini, yogurt and lemon juice in a bowl with the olive oil and garlic. Season with salt and pepper and whisk together.

Place the cabbage, onion, parsley and coriander/cilantro leaves in a large bowl, pour the dressing over the top and toss together well.

Heat a glug of rapeseed/canola oil in a large frying pan over a medium heat and, when hot, add the chicken escalopes. Cook for about 3 minutes on each side until the chicken is cooked all the way through. Leave to rest.

Slice the ciabatta rolls in half and rub a little olive oil over the cut sides. Place the cut sides down in the same frying pan and cook for 1–2 minutes until golden.

To assemble the sandwiches, start with a layer of salad leaves, then 2 chicken escalopes, followed by a generous amount of slaw and lastly the top half of the ciabatta. Repeat with the remaining ingredients.

TURKEY RAGU WITH PAPPARDELLE

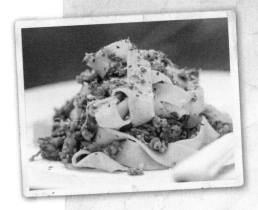

Festive recipes aside, there are relatively few dishes that make the most of turkey. Relatively inexpensive, turkey is well suited to sauces and pasta dishes such as in this recipe, or to bakes like lasagne and moussaka.

Heat a little rapeseed/canola oil in a saucepan and add the onion, celery and garlic. Cook for 5 minutes, until translucent and softened but not coloured.

Stir in the tomato purée/paste, oregano and parsley and cook for 1 minute, then add the turkey. Cook the meat for 5 minutes until it starts to colour and is sealed, stirring all the time and breaking up the meat if needed.

Add the tomatoes and stock and season with salt and pepper. Bring to the boil, turn down the heat, and simmer for 15 minutes. Add 1 tablespoon balsamic vinegar and cook for a further 5 minutes. Check the seasoning, adding more salt, pepper or balsamic vinegar to taste.

Meanwhile, bring a large pan of salted water to the boil. Add the pappardelle and cook for 8–10 minutes until al dente. Drain the pasta, return to the pan and toss a little olive oil through the pasta. Add the turkey ragu to the pappardelle and mix thoroughly together over a low heat.

Use a pair of tongs to pile the pasta onto plates, and top with a little Parmesan grated over and extra chopped parsley.

READY IN 40 MINUTES

SERVES 4

rapeseed/canola oil, for cooking

1 onion, chopped

1 celery stalk, finely chopped

1 garlic clove, crushed

2 tsp tomato purée/paste

1 tsp dried oregano

handful of chopped parsley, plus extra for sprinkling

450g/1lb minced/ground turkey

800g/1lb 12oz/3½ cups canned chopped tomatoes

200ml/7fl oz/¾ cup chicken or vegetable stock

1–2 tbsp balsamic vinegar

400g/14oz pappardelle

sea salt and freshly ground black pepper

olive oil, for drizzling

grated Parmesan cheese, to serve

NOTE: Minced/ground pork, chicken or veal all work well in place of turkey in this recipe.

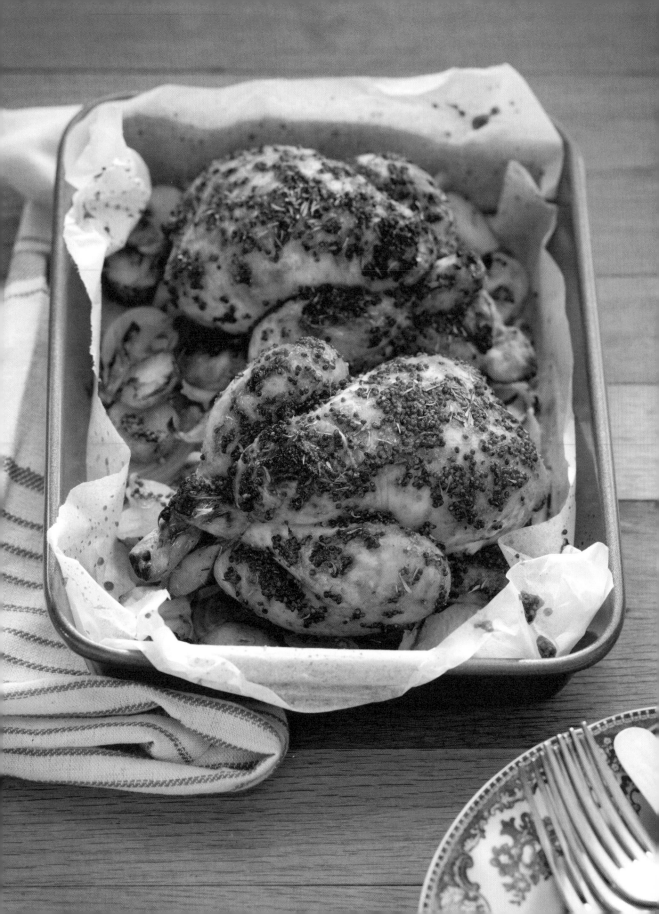

HONEY AND MUSTARD-GLAZED POUSSIN

Super-simple, I'm sure most people have tried a version of this classic flavour combination served with chicken. The beauty of poussin is the speedy cooking time, making this a great option for a quick meal during the week.

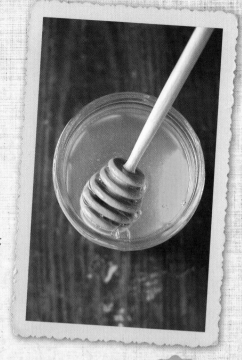

Preheat the oven to 200°C/400°F/gas 6.

In a small bowl, combine the mustard, honey, soy sauce, thyme and 1 tablespoon of the olive oil. Stir well and add a little salt and pepper.

Slice the potatoes very finely using a mandoline or the single blade on a box grater. Tip the sliced potatoes and onion into a roasting tray with the remaining olive oil and some more salt and pepper. Toss together and spread out evenly over the base of the tray.

Rub the honey and mustard mixture all over the skin of the poussin, including the legs. Place the birds on top of the onions and potatoes and roast in the oven for 35 minutes. Test that the poussin are cooked through by pulling gently at one of the legs, which should come away easily.

Cut the birds in half with a pair of scissors and serve on the bone, or carve as you would a chicken. Serve with the potatoes and onions, green salad and perhaps some homemade Grainy Mustard Mayonnaise.

READY IN 40 MINUTES

SERVES 4

2 tbsp wholegrain mustard

1 tbsp runny honey

1 tbsp soy sauce

2 tsp fresh thyme, chopped

2 tbsp olive oil

2 potatoes (about 300g/10½oz), peeled

1 onion, sliced

2 poussin

sea salt and freshly ground black pepper

green salad, to serve

Grainy Mustard Mayonnaise (see page 169), to serve (optional)

GUINEA FOWL WITH MARSALA, LENTILS AND SPINACH

Earthy, rich and reminiscent of late autumn evenings, a version of this dish used to be a favourite on my dinner party menus. This recipe uses guinea fowl breasts but you could use a whole jointed bird instead; just be sure to check the legs are cooked all the way through before serving.

SERVES 4

READY IN **40** MINUTES

140g/5oz/¾ cup dried Puy lentils

200g/7oz/4 cups spinach leaves

rapeseed/canola oil or butter, for cooking

4 guinea fowl breasts (skin on)

115g/4oz fresh shiitake mushrooms, roughly chopped

1 garlic clove, crushed

4 thyme sprigs

115ml/4fl oz/½ cup Marsala

170ml/5½fl oz/⅔ cup chicken stock

sea salt and freshly ground black pepper

Tip the lentils into a saucepan and cover with water. Add a little salt, bring to the boil and simmer gently for 10–15 minutes until they're cooked through but still retain a little bite.

Meanwhile, wash the spinach and place in another pan over a medium heat. Cover with a lid and cook for 2 minutes until the leaves have wilted. Tip into a colander and drain well, squeezing out as much moisture as you can.

Heat a little oil or butter in a large casserole dish. Season the guinea fowl breasts with salt and pepper and add them to the pan skin-side down. Cook for 5 minutes until the skin has turned golden brown. Turn them over and cook for another minute. Remove from the pan and leave to one side.

Add a little more oil or butter to the same pan and add the mushrooms, garlic and thyme and fry for 5 minutes until softened. Tip the cooked lentils into the pan, stir well and then pour in the Marsala. Simmer for 2 minutes until the liquid has been absorbed and then add the stock and cooked spinach. Stir well and season before returning the guinea fowl breasts to the pan, pushing them down gently into the lentils. Place a lid on the pan and simmer gently for 10 minutes.

Check the guinea fowl is cooked all the way through before serving.

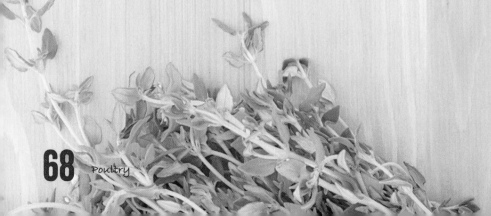

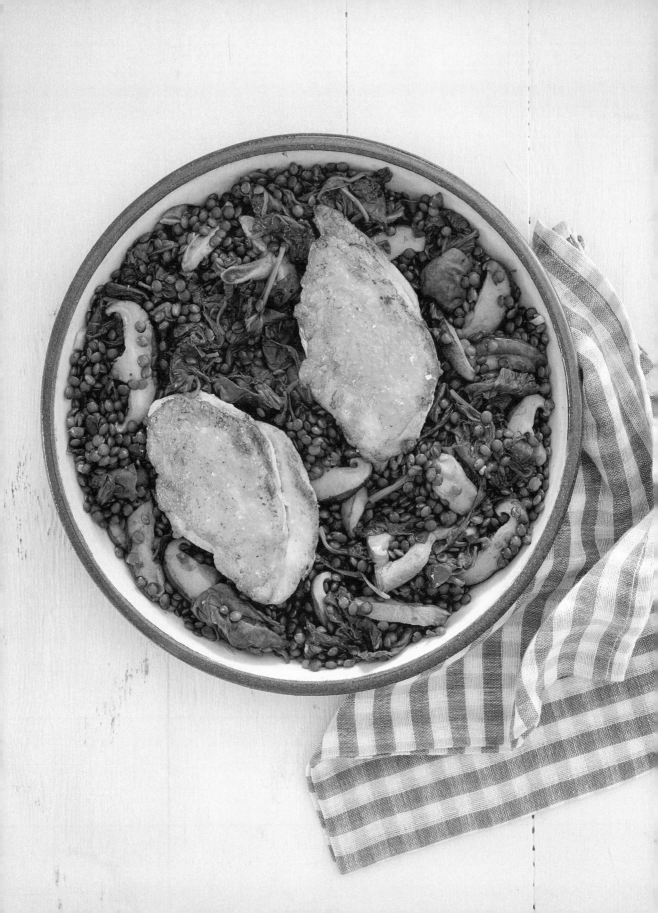

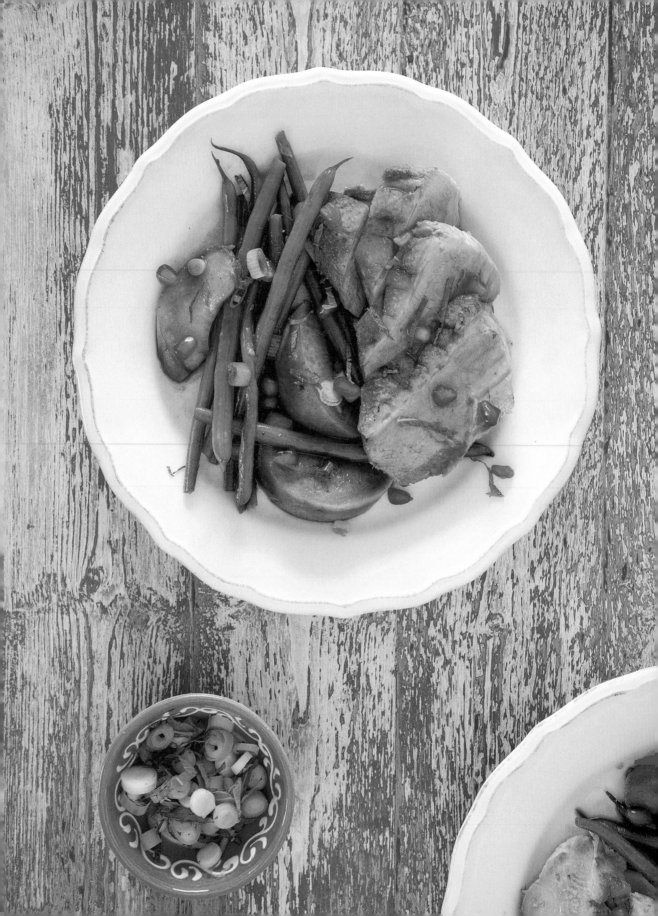

DUCK BREASTS WITH PEACHES AND BALSAMIC VINEGAR

Duck is a wonderful meat which isn't used as much as it should be. Although more expensive than other poultry, it's worth the price for an occasional treat. This sweet and piquant sauce is quick to put together and a complement to the gaminess of the bird.

Preheat the oven to 190°C/375°F/gas 5.

Using a very sharp knife, score the skin of the duck breasts in a diagonal direction being careful not to cut through to the meat. Turn the duck breast and score in the opposite direction so you end up with a criss-cross effect.

Place the duck breasts in a cold frying pan, skin-side down. Place the pan over a medium-high heat and fry for 6–8 minutes until the skin is golden and crispy (you do not need to add any oil as the duck contains enough fat). Flip over and cook on the flesh side for 1 minute. Lift out into a baking pan and cook in the oven for 7–10 minutes, depending on how rare you like your duck. Rest for a few minutes before serving.

Meanwhile, heat a pan of salted water until boiling and cook the beans for 2–3 minutes until just cooked. Rinse under cold running water, drain, and leave to one side.

Discard most of the fat in the pan you cooked the duck in, leaving about 2 tablespoons for the sauce. Return the pan to the heat and, once sizzling, add the spring onions/scallions and star anise. Fry for 2 minutes and then add the peaches. Cook for another minute, stirring well before adding the pomegranate juice and balsamic vinegar.

Turn the heat up and simmer for 3–4 minutes to reduce the sauce to a syrupy consistency. Add a little salt and pepper and taste the sauce; if it's a little sharp, add a squeeze of honey. Gently stir in the cooked beans.

Slice the duck, pouring any meat juices into the sauce, and serve with the peaches, beans and sauce spooned on top. Scatter some mint leaves and pomegranate seeds on top of each plate.

READY IN **30** MINUTES

SERVES 4

4 duck breasts (skin on)

110g/4oz fine/French beans

2 spring onions/scallions, sliced

1 star anise

2 ripe peaches, pitted and sliced into wedges

55ml/2oz/¼ cup pomegranate juice

55ml/2oz/¼ cup balsamic vinegar

squeeze of honey (optional)

sea salt and freshly ground black pepper

few mint leaves, shredded, for sprinkling

pomegranate seeds, to serve

PHEASANT, COCONUT AND TAMARIND CURRY

Pheasant lends itself really well to mild spices and is especially good paired with the tangy freshness of tamarind. This is a great way to enliven a much under-used meat. Serve with steamed wild rice and fine green beans.

SERVES 4

READY IN 30 MINUTES

2 tbsp rapeseed/canola oil, for cooking

1 onion, finely sliced

1 green pepper, sliced

1 green chilli, finely chopped

2cm/¾in piece of root ginger, peeled and grated

1 garlic clove, finely chopped

2 tsp yellow mustard seeds

1 tsp tomato purée/paste

1 tsp ground turmeric

4 pheasant breasts (each about 125g/4½oz), cut into bite-size pieces

2 tbsp tamarind paste

400ml/14fl oz/1⅔ cups coconut milk

1 tbsp soy sauce

squeeze of lime juice

sea salt and freshly ground black pepper

handful of coriander/cilantro leaves, for sprinkling

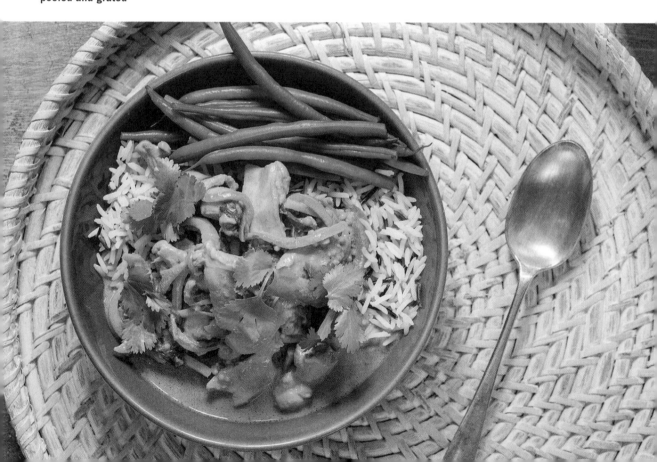

NOTE: Pheasant meat is delicate and doesn't contain much fat so it can dry out easily during cooking. Be careful to simmer the curry gently, rather than boil, and try a piece after 5 minutes to see if it's cooked through; it may not need the full 10 minutes cooking time.

If pheasant isn't readily available then you can use chicken breasts instead; they will still give you a zesty, piquant supper.

Heat the oil in a large frying pan over a medium-high heat and add the onion and pepper. Cook for 5 minutes, stirring occasionally, until the vegetables are soft and have taken on a little colour at the edges. Add the chilli, ginger and garlic and cook for a further 2 minutes.

Stir in the mustard seeds, tomato purée/paste and turmeric, adding a little more oil if the vegetables are dry and catching on the bottom of the pan.

Add the pheasant and stir well for 3–4 minutes to seal the meat.

Next, add the tamarind paste and coconut milk and stir through. Bring to a simmer and cook very gently for 5–10 minutes until the pheasant pieces are cooked through. Stir in the soy sauce, add a squeeze of lime juice and add salt and pepper if needed. Scatter over the coriander/cilantro.

Serve with rice and steamed green beans. Lime pickle is wonderful with this too.

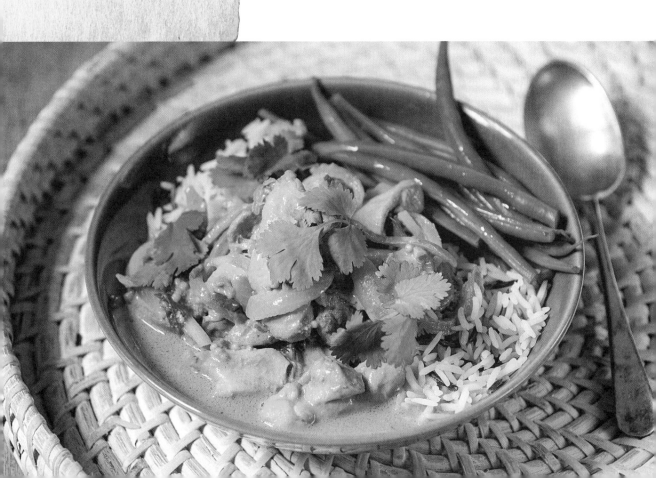

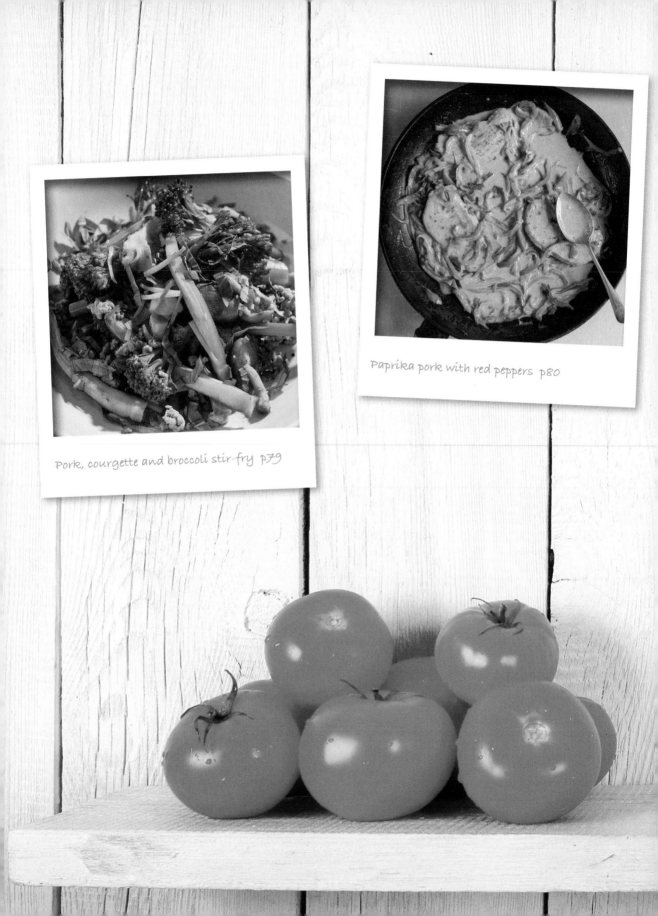

Pork, courgette and broccoli stir-fry p79

Paprika pork with red peppers p80

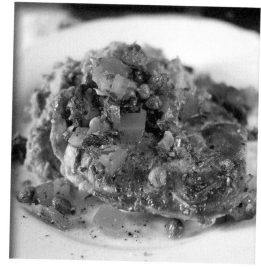

Lamb with bashed peas and tomato & mint salsa p99

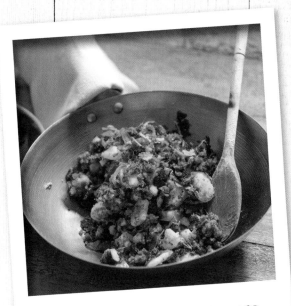

Corned beef hash with roast tomatoes p92

MEAT

PORK CHOPS BAKED WITH POTATOES AND APPLES

This easy meal almost feels like an indulgent Sunday roast, as the potatoes, rosemary and apple sizzle happily in the oven, filling the kitchen with mouth-watering aromas, but you can make it very quickly during the week. Buy the best-quality pork chops you can find. Cooked first in a hot pan until the fat is crisp and golden, then finished in the oven, the chops will stay tender and moist in the middle. This is very good with a bottle of cider.

SERVES 4

READY IN 40 MINUTES

1 large onion, sliced

4 potatoes, cut into wedges

2 rosemary stalks, leaves only

rapeseed/canola oil, for cooking

4 pork loin chops

115ml/4fl oz/½ cup vegetable stock

115ml/4fl oz/½ cup cider

2 apples, sliced and cored

sea salt and freshly ground black pepper

Preheat the oven to 190°C/375°F/gas 5.

Toss the onion and potato wedges in a bowl with the rosemary, a little salt and pepper and a little oil. Spread them out in a deep roasting tray or oven-proof dish and roast at the top of the oven for 20 minutes.

Meanwhile, heat a little oil in a frying pan and once hot, add the pork chops. Cook for about 3 minutes on each side until they turn nicely golden. Remove from the pan and leave to one side. Pour the stock and cider into the pan, turn up the heat and simmer for 3–4 minutes to reduce the liquid to a syrupy consistency.

After the potatoes and onions have been in the oven for 20 minutes, add the apples to the tray or dish and mix well. Lay the pork chops on top of the vegetables and pour the syrupy pan juices over everything.

Return the tray or dish to the oven and cook for another 12–15 minutes, or until the pork is cooked through.

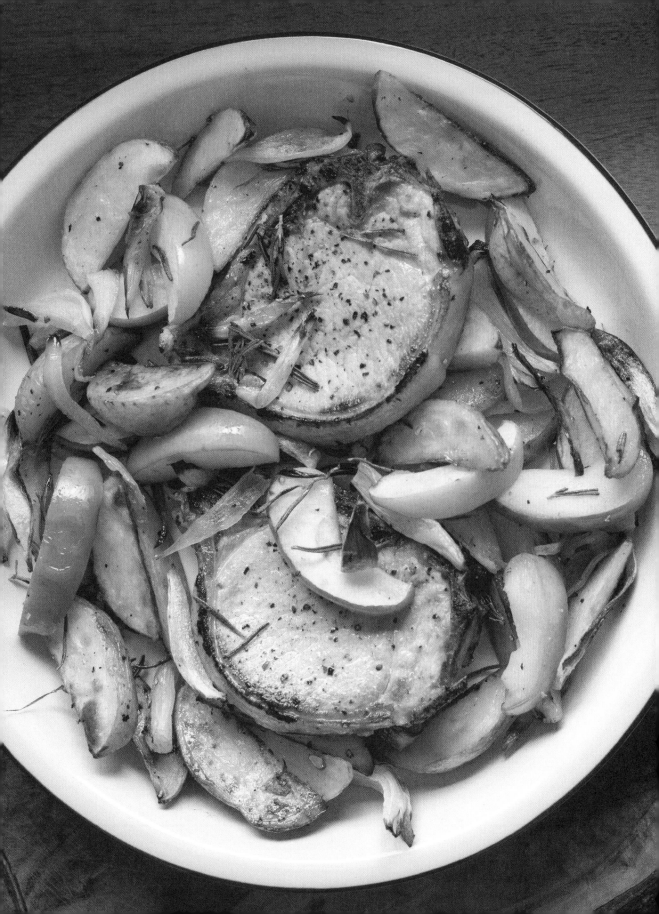

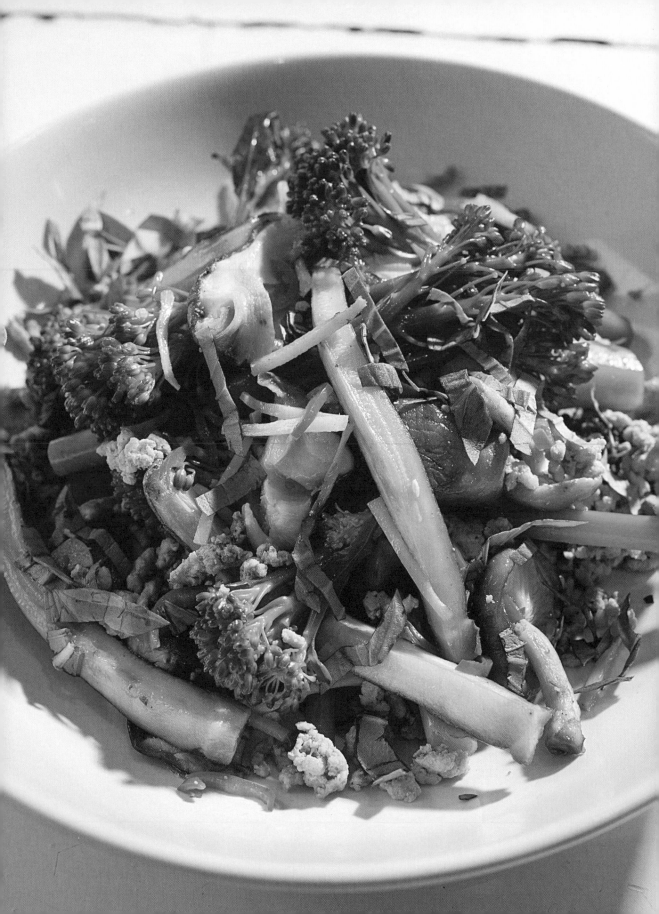

PORK, COURGETTE AND BROCCOLI STIR-FRY

This takes only minutes to throw together and makes for a light and healthy after-work meal. Turkey or beef work equally well if you want a variation from pork.

Bring a pan of salted water to the boil and cook the broccoli/broccolini for about 3 minutes until just tender. Drain then cool under cold running water. Leave to one side.

Heat 2 tablespoons of sesame oil in a large wok or frying pan and once hot, add the pork. Break it up with a spoon or spatula, stirring continuously for about 5 minutes until it turns opaque. Add the soy sauce, mix well and cook for a further minute. Tip the pork into a dish and leave to one side.

Add a little more oil to the pan and when hot, add the courgettes/zucchini, spring onions/scallions and mushrooms and cook for 2–3 minutes, shaking the pan and stir-frying the ingredients over the heat. Add the chilli, garlic and ginger and stir-fry for another 2 minutes before adding the broccoli/broccolini.

Return the pork to the pan, stir thoroughly and add the Thai basil and lime juice. Taste, adding some black pepper and extra soy sauce if needed. Serve with steamed rice or udon noodles.

READY IN 20 MINUTES

SERVES 4

285g/10oz Tenderstem broccoli/broccolini

sesame oil, for cooking

450g/1lb minced/ground pork

4 tbsp soy sauce, plus extra to taste

285g/10oz baby courgettes/zucchini, sliced into thin lengths

bunch of spring onions/scallions, sliced

200g/7oz shiitake mushrooms, sliced

1 red chilli, finely chopped

2 garlic cloves, crushed

5cm/2in piece of root ginger, peeled and grated

12 Thai basil leaves (or coriander/cilantro if you can't find this), shredded

juice of ½ lime

sea salt and freshly ground black pepper

steamed rice or udon noodles, to serve

PAPRIKA PORK WITH RED PEPPERS

SERVES 4

rapeseed/canola oil, for cooking

4 pork chops or escalopes

1 onion, sliced

2 red peppers, deseeded and sliced

1 garlic clove, sliced

2 tsp paprika

1 tsp tomato purée/paste

200ml/7fl oz/¾ cup chicken or vegetable stock

200ml/7fl oz/¾ cup crème fraîche

handful of parsley, chopped, plus extra for sprinkling

sea salt and freshly ground black pepper

mashed potatoes or steamed rice and green vegetables, to serve

Lightly spiced and satisfyingly creamy, this pork recipe needs only a handful of ingredients. This is my interpretation of a classic flavour combination, the addition of sliced red peppers adding a little more depth and texture.

Heat 1 tablespoon of oil in a large frying pan and fry the pork chops or escalopes for 2 minutes on each side until lightly golden brown. Remove to a plate.

Add a little more oil to the pan and add the onion, red peppers and garlic. Cook over a medium heat for about 10 minutes until soft and translucent, stirring every so often.

Stir the paprika and tomato purée/paste into the vegetables and then pour over the stock. Return the pork to the pan, bring to a simmer and cook for 5 minutes until the sauce is slightly syrupy. Add the crème fraîche, season with salt and pepper and simmer for 2 minutes before stirring in the parsley.

Serve with a little extra parsley sprinkled over, and mashed potatoes or steamed rice and green vegetables.

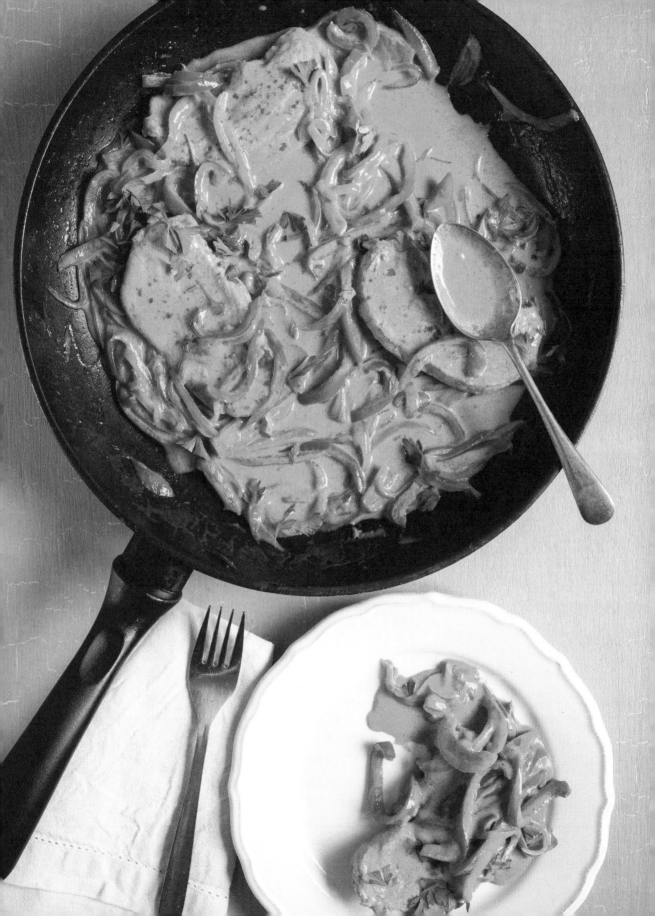

PORK FILLET WITH GINGER AND SOY

READY IN 30 MINUTES

SERVES 4

juice and zest of 1 large orange

6 tbsp dark soy sauce

1½ tbsp brown sugar

2 garlic cloves, crushed

2cm/¾in piece of root ginger, peeled and grated

2 pork fillets

2 tbsp rapeseed/canola oil

3 pak choi/bok choy

sea salt and freshly ground black pepper

sesame oil, for drizzling

1 tbsp sesame seeds, toasted, to serve (optional)

This tangy sauce takes on an almost caramel flavour once reduced, which really lifts the pork. I serve it with a pile of steamed rice and greens like pak choi/bok choy.

Preheat the oven to 200°C/400°F/gas 6.

Combine the orange juice, soy sauce, sugar, garlic and ginger in a small saucepan and heat gently, stirring, until the sugar has dissolved. Add the orange zest and stir in. Leave to one side.

Slice each pork fillet in half, trimming and discarding any thick pieces of fat or tough membrane, so you have 4 pieces. Season each with a little salt and pepper.

Heat the rapeseed/canola oil in a frying pan and, when hot, cook the pork for 2 minutes on each side until browned. Place in a roasting tray and roast for 12–15 minutes until cooked through.

Meanwhile, pour the soy and orange mixture into the pan in which you browned the pork, stirring to incorporate any residue from the bottom of the pan. Bring to a simmer and cook the mixture for about 5 minutes until you have a thick, sticky sauce.

Take the pork out of the oven and leave it to rest while you steam the pak choi/bok choy for 5 minutes.

Slice the pork and pour any extra juices into the sauce and mix well. Dress the greens with a little sesame oil and serve alongside the pork with the sauce spooned over the top and sprinkled with some toasted sesame seeds, if you like.

SPICED SAUSAGE-STUFFED ROMANO PEPPERS

A great way to use up leftover rice and to add interest to a pack of sausages, these stuffed peppers are very simple to prepare. You could also keep one for a packed lunch. Romano peppers are the long peppers available in most supermarkets; they have a lovely sweet flavour, but if you can't find them then normal peppers will work as well.

SERVES 4

2 tbsp rapeseed/canola oil, for cooking

1 onion, finely chopped

1 garlic clove, crushed

1 courgette/zucchini, finely chopped

6 pork sausages

1 tsp tomato purée/paste

1 tsp dried oregano

1 tsp chilli powder

200g/7oz/2 cups cooked rice

2 tbsp finely chopped parsley

4 Romano peppers

55g/2oz Parmesan cheese, grated

sea salt and freshly ground black pepper

Preheat the oven to 200°C/400°F/gas 6.

Heat the oil in a frying pan over a medium heat. Add the onion and garlic and fry for 5 minutes until softened. Add the courgette/zucchini and cook for another 2 minutes.

Squeeze the sausage meat out of its casings straight into the pan, breaking up the meat with a wooden spoon over the heat. Continue to cook the mixture gently for 5 minutes, stirring often, until the sausage meat is slightly browned and cooked through.

Stir in the tomato purée/paste, oregano and chilli powder and cook for 1 minute before stirring in the rice and parsley. Season with salt and pepper.

Cut the peppers in half lengthways, leaving the stems intact if you can, and cut out the pith and seeds. Divide the sausage mixture between the peppers and sprinkle the Parmesan over. Place on a baking sheet and bake at the top of the oven for 20 minutes until the peppers are soft and the top of the filling is nicely golden.

CHORIZO, LEEK & CIDER-BRAISED LENTILS

There is a classic Spanish tapas dish of fat chorizo slices braised in cider, which is where the idea for this dish came from, made more substantial with the addition of lentils. The sliced leeks soak up the chorizo's rich oil, which seeps from the sausage as it cooks, while the sweet cider bubbles away to leave a syrupy sauce for the lentils. Served with chunks of bread torn from the loaf, you couldn't have a more rustic, autumnal supper.

SERVES 4

READY IN 30 MINUTES

170g/6oz cooking chorizo

2 leeks, finely sliced

2 garlic cloves, crushed

rapeseed/canola oil, for cooking, if needed

1 heaped tsp paprika

400g/14oz cooked Puy lentils

2 tbsp chopped parsley

400ml/14fl oz/1¾ cups cider

2 tbsp white wine vinegar

sea salt and freshly ground black pepper

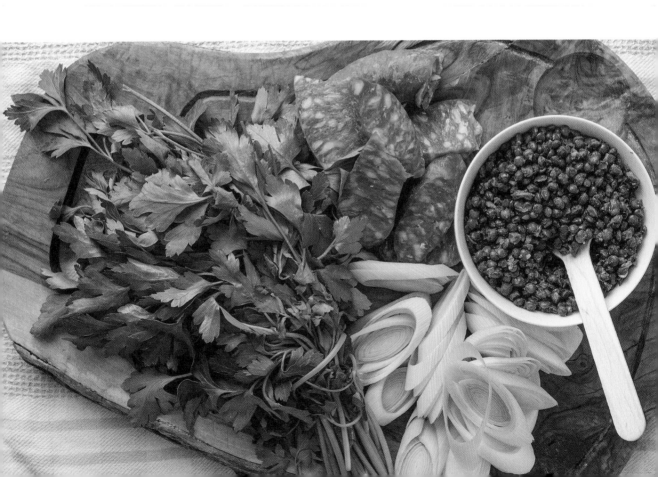

NOTE: Choose soft, uncooked chorizo sausage for this recipe. The firmer, drier cured version won't give you the same depth of flavour or release such delicious spicy oil as it cooks.

Pouches of pre-cooked lentils are useful to keep in the cupboard and work well in this recipe.

Slice the chorizo on the angle into pieces about 5mm/¼in thick. Heat a deep frying pan, add the chorizo, and fry for 5 minutes over a medium heat until it releases red oil into the pan and starts to darken at the edges.

Add the leeks and garlic, stir well and cook for another 10 minutes until the leeks have wilted and softened. Add a glug of oil if the mixture seems too dry.

Stir in the paprika, lentils and half of the parsley and then pour in the cider. Bring to the boil, then turn the heat down to a simmer and leave to gently bubble for 10 minutes until the lentils have absorbed most of the liquid. If the mixture seems a little too dry, add a touch more cider.

Stir in the vinegar, season with salt and pepper and serve with the remaining parsley scattered over the top.

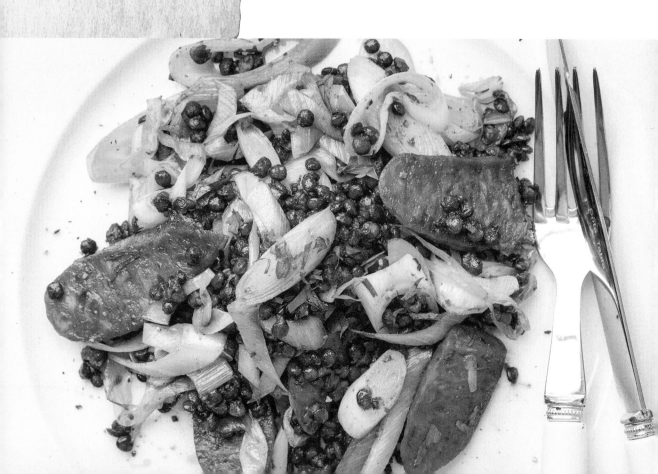

FIG, PROSCIUTTO AND GORGONZOLA CROUTES

This recipe, given to me by a good friend and fellow cook, Bella Thomas-Ferrand, sings of indulgent Italian eating, both with its classic flavours and ease of preparation. A friendly greengrocer will find you figs, but failing that, good supermarkets have them out of season. After a few days in the fruit bowl and the help of sticky balsamic caramel they will be delicious.

If sourdough isn't available then any good-quality crusty loaf will work, the chewier and more rustic the better.

SERVES 4

READY IN 15 MINUTES

6 tbsp balsamic vinegar

2 tbsp brown sugar

8 ripe figs

2 tbsp pine nuts

8 slices of sourdough bread

2 garlic cloves, peeled

extra virgin olive oil, for drizzling

8 slices of prosciutto

100g/3½oz Gorgonzola cheese, crumbled

handful of rocket/arugula

sea salt and freshly ground black pepper

Pour the vinegar into a small pan, add the brown sugar and heat gently. Once the sugar has dissolved, turn the heat up and simmer rapidly until the liquid is reduced and syrupy.

Slice the figs into quarters, vertically through their stalks, and place cut-side down in the balsamic syrup. Cook over a medium heat, with the syrup bubbling, for 1–2 minutes, then turn the fig quarters, spooning the liquid over the figs. Remove the figs to a small plate, then boil the remaining syrup until reduced to a thick glaze.

Meanwhile, toast the pine nuts in a small frying pan for 1–2 minutes until lightly coloured, then leave to one side. Toast the sourdough on both sides using a griddle/grill pan or alternatively under a grill/broiler. Rub the garlic cloves over the toasted bread, then drizzle with olive oil.

While the bread is still warm, top each slice with 2 slices of prosciutto, followed by the caramelized figs, Gorgonzola and a drizzle of both the balsamic glaze and some more extra virgin olive oil. Scatter over the rocket/arugula and pine nuts and grind over some salt and pepper.

NOTE: This recipe works well with any type of soft blue sheeps' or goats' cheese. I'd particularly recommend Lanark Blue made in central Scotland or, of course, Roquefort.

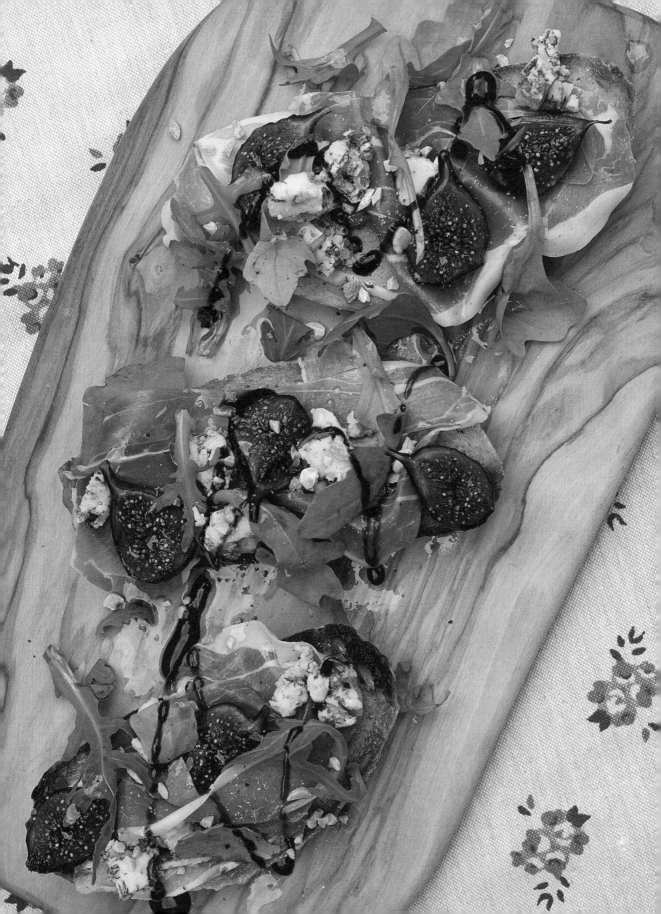

OPEN SERRANO HAM, GOATS' CHEESE AND SPINACH QUESADILLAS

READY IN **30** MINUTES

SERVES 4

200g/7oz/4 cups fresh spinach leaves

4 soft tortillas

olive or rapeseed/canola oil, for brushing

8–12 thin slices of Serrano ham

100g/3½oz soft goats' cheese (or any soft cheese)

8 jalapeño peppers, sliced

sea salt and freshly ground black pepper

tomato, avocado or sweetcorn salad, to serve

NOTE: You can experiment with any number of ingredients for this recipe; roasted peppers, chorizo, anchovies, chillies, olives, Parma ham/prosciutto or mozzarella would all work well.

For anyone avoiding wheat or gluten, try using corn tortillas or gluten-free wraps, which are available in most supermarkets.

Light, crisp and ready to eat in no more time than it takes for your grill/broiler to warm, these quesadillas will shoot to the top of your weekday favourites. I first had a version in La Bodega Negra, a restaurant in London, where they arrive as an appetizer. Here, with a whole tortilla each and served with an avocado, sweetcorn or tomato salad, you won't need much else.

Preheat your grill/broiler to its highest setting.

Throw the spinach leaves into a large pan with a sprinkling of water, cover with a lid and cook for 2 minutes until the leaves have just wilted. Drain and then squeeze out as much excess water as you can.

Brush the tortillas with oil on both sides and lay them flat on a board. Cover each with 2–3 slices of Serrano ham and then divide the cooked spinach between them. Crumble the goats' cheese into the gaps and lastly scatter over the jalapeños. Season with salt and pepper.

Place a large frying pan over a medium heat and brush the base with a little more oil. Place a tortilla into the pan and fry for 2–3 minutes until the edges are slightly crisp and the cheese begins to melt. Place the pan under the hot grill/broiler for 1–2 minutes until the cheese starts to bubble and turn golden. Repeat with the remaining tortillas, keeping the cooked ones warm in a low oven until you've finished cooking.

Serve with sliced tomato, avocado or sweetcorn salad, or a combination of all three.

TOULOUSE SAUSAGE WITH FENNEL AND LENTILS

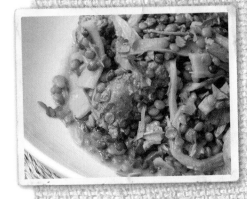

This wholesome supper works best with rich Toulouse sausages, which are flavoured with bacon, wine and herbs. Most butchers and supermarkets stock a version of these but if you don't have any luck finding them, use a good-quality pork sausage and add some chopped smoked bacon to the pan at the beginning of the recipe.

Twist each sausage in the middle to form 2 smaller sausages, then cut with a pair of scissors so you have 16 small sausages.

Heat a little oil in a casserole pan and cook the sausages for 5–6 minutes until browned all over. Remove to a plate and leave to one side.

Add a little more oil to the same pan and, when hot, add the carrot and fennel. Fry for 5 minutes until softened and slightly coloured. Add the garlic, tomato purée/paste and rosemary to the pan and cook for 1–2 minutes.

Return the sausages to the pan, followed by the lentils, parsley, bay leaf and some salt and pepper. Pour in half the stock, bring to the boil, turn the heat down and simmer for 10–15 minutes covered with a lid. Stir every so often, adding the rest of the stock as needed to stop the mixture drying out.

Taste to check the seasoning and serve with some wilted spinach or steamed green beans.

READY IN 40 MINUTES

SERVES 4

8 Toulouse sausages

rapeseed/canola oil, for frying

1 large carrot, peeled and finely chopped

1 fennel bulb, finely sliced

1 garlic clove, crushed

1 tsp tomato purée/paste

2 tsp dried rosemary

800g/1lb 12oz cooked Puy lentils

handful of fresh parsley, roughly chopped, plus extra for sprinkling

1 bay leaf

250ml/9fl oz/1 cup chicken stock

sea salt and freshly ground black pepper

wilted spinach or steamed green beans, to serve

NOTE: If you have some leftover red wine lying around, add a glass or so in place of some of the stock.

BEEF STIR-FRY WITH GREEN PEPPERS

Taking a minute or two to make your own stir-fry sauce is really worth it. Not only will the result be fresher and tastier than anything you squeeze out of a sachet, but you can play around with the ingredients and adjust the seasonings to suit your own tastes. To this quite basic recipe, you could also add black-eyed beans, mangetout/snow peas, mushrooms or pak choi/bok choy in place of, or as well as, the vegetables listed. Don't worry if you don't have a wok, just use a large frying pan; the key is to cook quickly over a high heat without the ingredients being crowded.

READY IN 20 MINUTES

SERVES 4

1 heaped tsp cornflour/cornstarch

3 tbsp soy sauce

3 tbsp mirin (rice wine)

rapeseed/canola oil, for cooking

bunch of spring onions/scallions, sliced

2 green peppers, deseeded and sliced

2 garlic cloves, crushed

700g/1lb 9oz rump steak, sliced into strips

150ml/5fl oz/²⁄₃ cup stock

5 tbsp oyster sauce

3 tbsp sweet chilli sauce

2 tsp sesame seeds, toasted, to serve (optional)

steamed rice or noodles, to serve

Place the cornflour/cornstarch in a small bowl and stir in the soy sauce and mirin until you have a smooth paste.

Heat 2 tablespoons of oil over a high heat and, when very hot, add the spring onions/scallions, peppers and garlic. Cook for 4–5 minutes, stirring often, until the vegetables are tender and slightly golden at the edges, but still have a bit of bite. Tip out of the pan and leave to one side.

Add a little more oil to the pan and, when hot, add the beef. Cook for 3–4 minutes, stirring all of the time until the meat is cooked and has taken on some colour.

Take the pan off the heat and add the cornflour/cornstarch mixture, followed by the stock, oyster sauce and sweet chilli sauce. Return to the heat and bring to a simmer for 1–2 minutes until the sauce thickens. Add a little more stock if the sauce is too thick. Return the vegetables to the pan and stir to heat everything through.

Serve with a sprinkling of toasted sesame seeds, if you like, and some steamed rice or noodles.

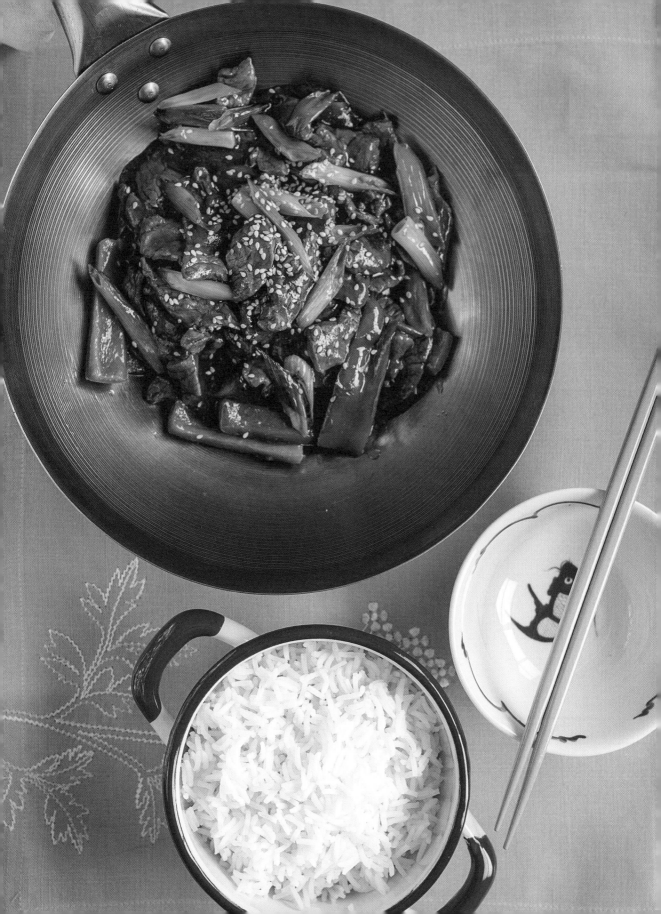

CORNED BEEF HASH WITH ROAST TOMATOES

This store-cupboard supper is real after-work comfort food. With hot English mustard and plenty of Worcestershire sauce to sharpen the flavours, it's a lot more satisfying and flavourful than its reputation would suggest. If you're really hungry, serve topped with a poached egg.

SERVES 4

READY IN 40 MINUTES

4 large tomatoes, halved

2 tbsp extra virgin olive oil

4 medium white potatoes (about 400g/14oz), peeled and chopped into cubes

rapeseed/canola oil, for cooking

1 large onion, finely sliced

340g/12oz corned beef, cut into 1cm/½in chunks

2 tsp English mustard

1 tbsp Worcestershire sauce

handful of parsley, roughly chopped

sea salt and freshly ground black pepper

4 eggs, poached (optional)

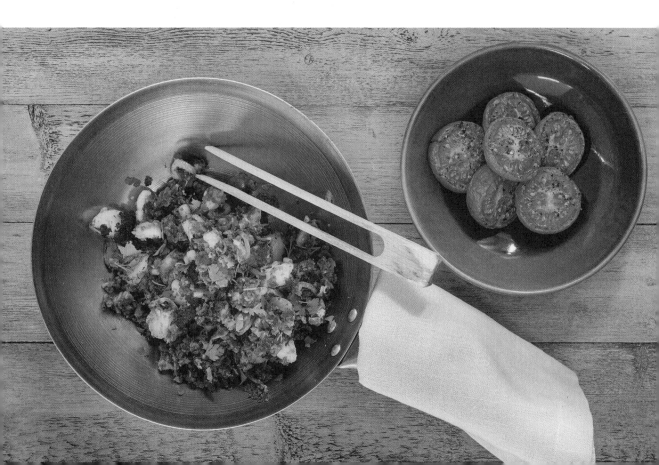

NOTE: Poaching eggs is one of those tasks new cooks are a little fearful of, but once you've got the hang of it they're very versatile and really not as tricky as you might think. The key is to find the freshest eggs you can.

To poach an egg, bring a pan of water to the boil, making sure you have a water depth of at least 10cm/4in. Add 1 tbsp white wine vinegar and reduce to a simmer. Crack a fresh egg into a cup, gently swirl the water, then pour the egg into the middle of the pan. After a few seconds, the shape of the egg will set. Cook for 4–5 minutes before removing the egg with a slotted spoon. Test if the egg is cooked to your liking by gently pressing on the yolk.

Preheat the oven to 200°C/400°F/gas 6.

Rub the cut sides of the tomatoes with the olive oil, season with salt and pepper and place in a baking pan, cut-sides up. Cook at the top of the oven for 15–20 minutes while you make the hash.

Put the potatoes in a large saucepan and cover with boiling water. Add a little salt, bring to the boil and simmer for 5 minutes. Drain and leave to one side.

Heat 2 tablespoons of rapeseed/canola oil in a large frying pan and, when almost smoking hot, add the onion. Fry for 5 minutes until softened and slightly golden. Add a little more oil to the pan, followed by the potatoes and fry for another 5 minutes, turning everything over in the oil every so often. The onions and potatoes should turn golden and slightly crisp at the edges.

Add the corned beef, stir together well, then fry for another 2–3 minutes, adding a little more oil if the mixture is dry. Add plenty of salt and pepper, along with the mustard, Worcestershire sauce and parsley. Taste and adjust the seasoning accordingly; you may prefer more mustard or Worcester sauce.

Serve with the roast tomatoes and a poached egg on top of each serving, if you like.

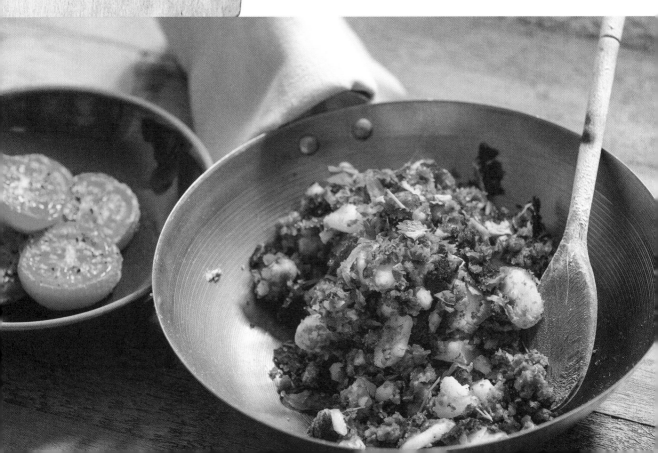

CHARGRILLED SIRLOIN STEAK WITH SALSA VERDE

A piquant herby sauce, salsa verde is a delicious accompaniment or dressing for meat, fish and vegetables. Here, it makes a quick and tasty partner to smoky, chargrilled steak. This recipe will leave you with some leftover sauce for a second meal or to use to dress potatoes or salads. You can either blitz everything in a blender, which takes no time at all, or chop the ingredients finely by hand.

SERVES 4

READY IN **15** MINUTES

4 sirloin steaks (each about 200g/7oz)

rocket/arugula, to serve

FOR THE SALSA VERDE

1 garlic clove

4 anchovy fillets

1 tsp Dijon mustard

1 tbsp red wine vinegar

1 tbsp capers

1 tbsp cornichons

2 large handfuls of parsley, leaves only

handful of mint leaves

handful of basil leaves

100ml/3½fl oz/scant ½ cup extra virgin olive oil, plus extra for drizzling

sea salt and freshly ground black pepper

To make the salsa verde, place the garlic in the bowl of a blender with the anchovies, mustard, vinegar, capers and cornichons and blitz to a paste; try to avoid any big chunks of garlic or cornichon in the finished sauce.

Add the parsley, mint, basil and olive oil and blitz again for 30 seconds or so until you have a coarse green sauce similar in texture to a thin pesto. Pour the salsa verde out into a bowl. Stir in some pepper and salt if it needs it; the salty anchovies and capers mean the salsa verde is unlikely to need too much. Leave to one side to allow the flavours to develop while you cook the steaks.

Heat a griddle/grill pan over a high heat. Rub a little olive oil and some salt and pepper into both sides of the steaks and when the pan is almost smoking add them to the pan, 2 at a time. (You don't want to overcrowd the pan by cooking 4 at once but if you have a huge griddle/grill plate or are using a barbecue, do cook them all at the same time.)

Cook the steaks for 2–3 minutes on each side, which is about right for medium-rare, depending on the thickness of the steaks. The best way to judge if they are cooked is to cut into one of the steaks and check that it looks right for your taste. Remove from the pan and leave to rest while you cook the remaining steaks.

Slice the steaks, then serve on a pile of rocket/arugula with the salsa verde drizzled over the top.

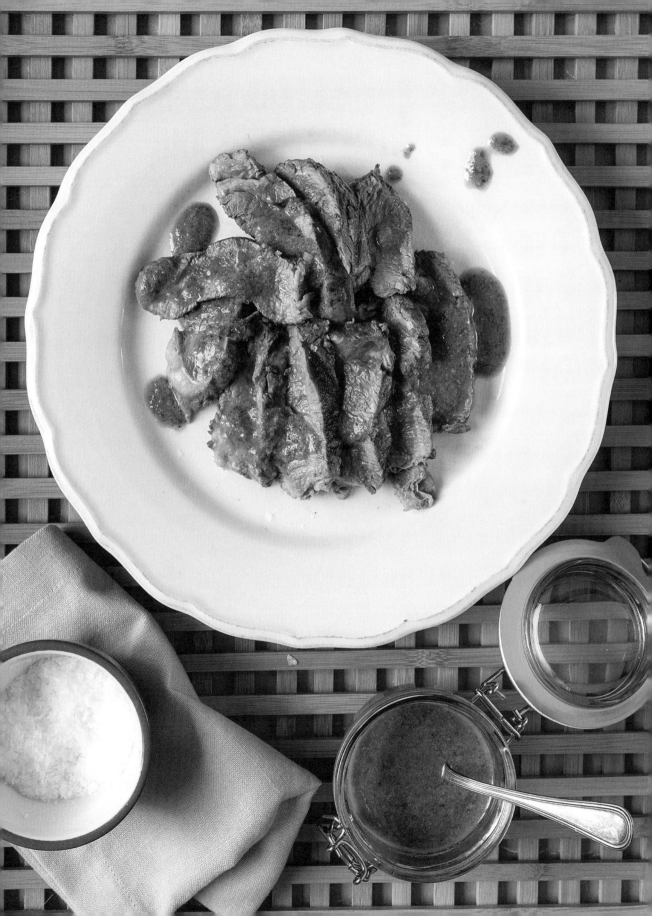

RUMP STEAK WRAPS WITH PEPPERS AND WATERCRESS SAUCE

SERVES 4

olive oil, for cooking

4 rump steaks (each about 200g/7oz)

3 peppers (choose either red, orange or yellow), deseeded and sliced into thin strips

1 red onion, sliced

1 garlic clove, sliced

8–12 tortilla wraps

sea salt and freshly ground black pepper

Watercress Sauce (see page 168), to serve

NOTE: If you're not a fan of watercress then you can make the dressing in exactly the same way but with rocket/ arugula or a mixture of any fresh herbs you have.

Rare juicy steak with peppery watercress and juicy, sweet peppers wrapped up in a floury tortilla – just as delicious at lunchtime or for a picnic as it is on your supper plate. I like to serve this with a green salad.

Preheat the oven to 200°C/400°F/gas 6.

Rub a little olive oil, salt and pepper into both sides of the steaks and leave to one side.

Place the peppers, onion and garlic in a roasting tray with a drizzle of olive oil. Season with salt and pepper, toss everything together and spread evenly over the base of the tray. Roast at the top of the oven for about 20 minutes until the vegetables are cooked and slightly golden at the edges.

Heat a griddle/grill pan or frying pan and, when very hot, add the steaks. Cook for just over 2 minutes on each side for rare steaks (depending on the thickness). If you prefer your steak cooked medium or well-done, then turn the heat down slightly and cook for 1–2 minutes longer on each side until cooked to your liking. You can cut into the steak to check the middle if you're unsure. Remove from the pan and leave to rest for a few minutes.

Heat the tortilla wraps according to the package directions. Decant the pepper and onion mixture into a serving dish and cut the steak into chunky slices. Serve the wraps, steak and vegetables at the table and drizzle the Watercress Sauce over the steak and peppers before wrapping up.

LAMB WITH BRAISED SPRING VEGETABLES

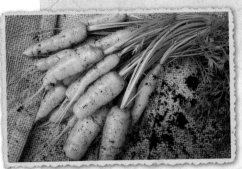

This classic French way to cook young vegetables is a lovely way to bring out their flavour while keeping them fresh and tender. Served with sliced, pink lamb, this makes a delicious evening meal.

Place the potatoes in a saucepan and cover with water. Add a little salt, bring to the boil, then turn down the heat, and simmer for about 10 minutes until tender. Drain, cool under cool running water and slice into 5mm/¼in discs.

Meanwhile, heat the olive oil and butter in a deep pan. Add the shallots and fry for 5 minutes. Add the carrots, garlic and thyme. Cook for another 2 minutes before pouring in the stock. Add a little salt and pepper, then bring to the boil, cover with a lid and simmer for 5 minutes.

Season the lamb with salt and pepper and heat a little rapeseed/canola oil in a frying pan. Add the lamb and cook for 2 minutes on each side until browned well, then lower the heat and cook for another 5–7 minutes, turning every so often to cook the meat evenly. Remove from the pan and leave to one side while you finish the vegetables.

Add the sliced potatoes, peas, broad/fava beans, mint and parsley to the shallots and carrots. Add a little more stock if the mixture looks dry and simmer for another 3 minutes or so, again covered with a lid, until the peas and beans are cooked. Season with salt and pepper to taste.

Slice the lamb fillets and serve on top of a pile of the braised vegetables, perhaps with a drizzle of mint sauce, if you like.

SERVES 4

READY IN **30** MINUTES

12–16 new/salad potatoes

2 tbsp olive oil

knob of butter

8 shallots, halved

16 baby carrots, halved lengthways

1 garlic clove, crushed

1 thyme sprig

225ml/8fl oz/1 cup chicken stock

4 lamb neck fillets (each about 180g/6¼oz)

rapeseed/canola oil, for frying

200g/7oz/1½ cups frozen peas

200g/7oz/1¾ cups frozen broad/fava beans

1 tbsp chopped mint

1 tbsp chopped parsley

sea salt and freshly ground black pepper

mint sauce, to serve (optional)

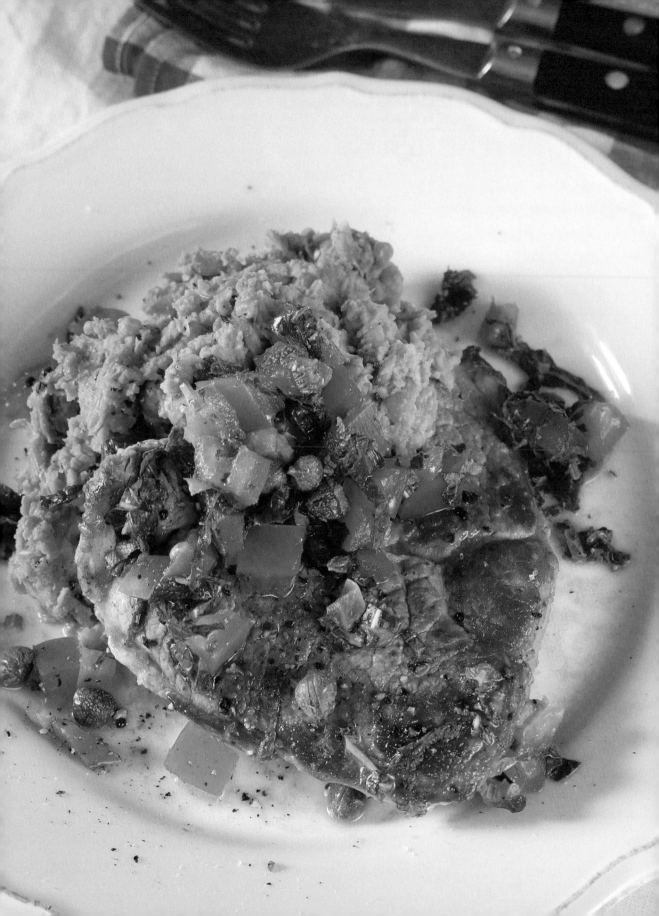

LAMB WITH BASHED PEAS AND TOMATO AND MINT SALSA

Inexpensive and widely available, leg steaks and gigot chops are often neglected cuts of lamb. Serving them with a fresh, tangy mint and tomato salsa really brings them to life without needing you to spend long in the kitchen. It also works as an accompaniment to a Sunday roast or lamb sausages. You can use any leftover salsa to dress salads.

Bring a pan of salted water to the boil and tip in the frozen peas. Bring back to the boil and simmer for 2 minutes, then drain.

Meanwhile, melt the butter in a small frying pan, add the spring onions/scallions and cook gently for 5 minutes until tender. Tip into a food processor or blender and add the peas, crème fraîche and half of the lemon juice. Blend using the pulse setting to a rough purée and season, adding the remaining lemon juice if needed. Leave to one side and keep warm while you cook the lamb and make the salsa.

Place the tomatoes in a small bowl with the capers and mint. Add the vinegar, olive oil and some black pepper. Stir well.

To cook the lamb, heat a little rapeseed/canola oil in a heavy frying pan. Season the lamb steaks or chops on both sides and add to the hot pan. Cook for 3–4 minutes on each side until golden brown and cooked through. The lamb should still be slightly pink in the middle but not bloody.

Rest the meat for 5 minutes and then serve with a large spoonful of the bashed peas and the salsa on top.

READY IN 20 MINUTES

SERVES 4

300g/10½oz/2 cups frozen peas

50g/1¾oz/¼ cup butter

6 spring onions/scallions, finely sliced

4 tbsp crème fraîche

juice of 1 lemon

4 tomatoes, diced

2 tbsp capers

3 tbsp mint leaves, finely shredded

2 tbsp white wine vinegar

4 tbsp extra virgin olive oil

rapeseed/canola oil, for cooking

4 lamb leg steaks or gigot chops (each about 140g/5oz)

sea salt and freshly ground black pepper

NOTE: Lamb steaks and chops also grill/broil beautifully. Preheat the grill/broiler to high, season the lamb as above, and cook for 3–4 minutes on each side before resting.

VENISON SAUSAGE, KALE AND RED WINE CASSEROLE

Venison sausages have found their way onto most supermarket shelves and make a leaner and healthier alternative to pork. Earthy and comforting, this quick casserole is lovely served with fluffy mashed potatoes or polenta/cornmeal.

READY IN 40 MINUTES

SERVES 4

rapeseed/canola oil, for frying

600g/1lb 5oz venison sausages

2 red onions, sliced

1 garlic clove, sliced

225g/8oz button mushrooms

2 tsp dried rosemary

300ml/10½fl oz/1¼ cups red wine

300ml/10½fl oz/1¼ cups beef stock

1 tbsp redcurrant jelly, plus extra to serve (optional)

1–2 tsp English mustard, to taste, plus extra to serve (optional)

1 tsp cornflour/cornstarch

3 large handfuls of kale, chopped

sea salt and freshly ground black pepper

Heat a little oil in a large casserole pan and, when hot, add the sausages. Cook for about 5 minutes until they are browned well all over. Add the onions, garlic and mushrooms to the pan. Stir well to coat the vegetables in the oil and cook for 7–10 minutes, stirring every so often, until the onion has softened and slightly browned. Add a little more oil if needed.

Add the rosemary, stir well and then pour in the red wine and stock, followed by the redcurrant jelly and mustard. Stir again, bring to the boil, then turn the heat down and leave to gently simmer for 15 minutes until the sausages are cooked through.

In a small cup, mix 1 tablespoon of water into the cornflour/cornstarch to form a lump-free paste. Take the pan off the heat and stir this into the sauce. Return the pan to the heat and add the kale. Place a lid on top of the pan and simmer for 2–3 minutes until the leaves have wilted. Stir well and season with salt and pepper and a little more mustard if needed. Serve with extra mustard and redcurrant jelly, if you like.

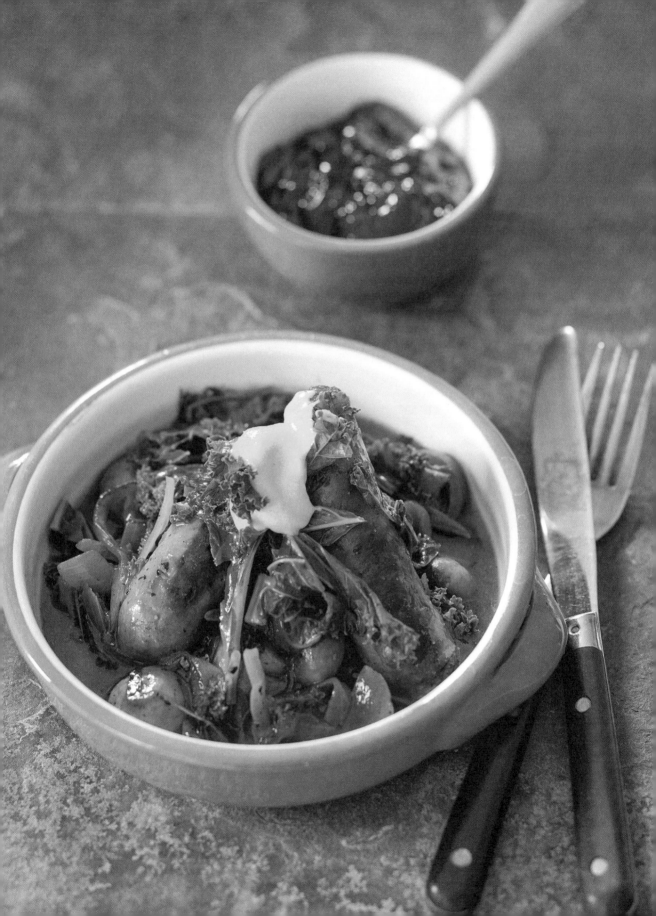

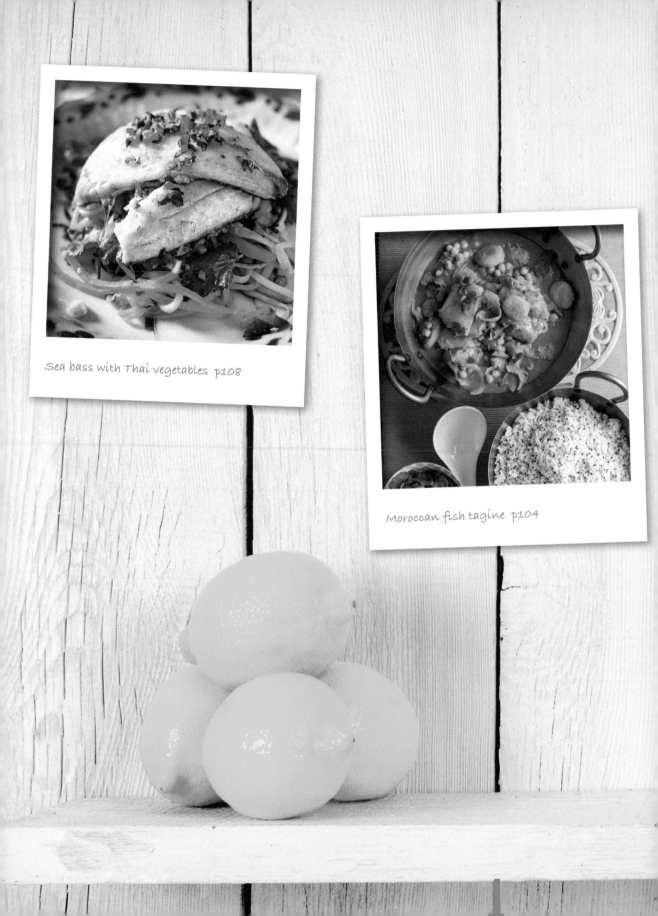

Sea bass with Thai vegetables p108

Moroccan fish tagine p104

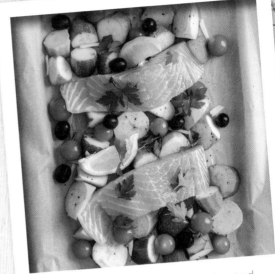

Garlic roast salmon with courgettes and olives p114

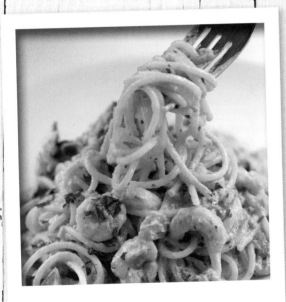

Spicy prawn and tomato spaghetti p122

FISH

MOROCCAN FISH TAGINE

SERVES 4

rapeseed/canola oil, for cooking

1 large onion, chopped

1 garlic clove, crushed

1 tsp tomato purée/paste

1 tsp ground turmeric

1 tsp ground cumin

1 tsp ground coriander

400g/14oz/1¾ cups canned chopped tomatoes

450ml/15fl oz/1¾ cups fish or vegetable stock

400g/14oz canned chickpeas, drained

3 strips of lemon peel

115g/4oz/¾ cup dried apricots or sultanas/golden raisins

4 firm white fish fillets, such as cod or haddock (each about 200g/7oz)

handful of coriander/cilantro leaves, chopped

sea salt and freshly ground black pepper

couscous, to serve (optional)

nigella (black onion) seeds, to serve (optional)

Meaty tagines, made with lamb or beef, are cooked slowly for hours giving them wonderful depth and tenderness, but this makes them impractical for most of us midweek. If you use fish or shellfish instead, you can have something ready in less than half an hour.

This is a mild, mellow tagine that can be spiced up with chilli or sweetened with honey. To this you can add olives, saffron, flaked/sliced almonds, green peppers or preserved lemons and if you can manage a moment or two of extra chopping, then use fresh plum tomatoes instead of canned. Try serving with a bowl of couscous or flatbreads and salad.

Heat a little oil in a large saucepan and add the onion and garlic. Cook for 5 minutes until softened but not coloured. Stir in the tomato purée/paste and turmeric, cumin and ground coriander and cook for 1 minute. Add the tomatoes, stock, chickpeas, lemon peel and apricots or sultanas/golden raisins. Bring to the boil, then turn down the heat and simmer for 15 minutes, stirring every so often.

Add some salt and pepper and stir in, then add the fish fillets to the tagine, gently pushing them down into the sauce. Continue to cook over a very low heat, so that the sauce is just simmering, for 5 minutes until the fish turns opaque and is cooked through. Meanwhile, if you want to serve couscous, cook according to the package directions.

Scatter the coriander/cilantro over the top of the tagine. Fluff up the couscous, if using, and scatter over a few nigella seeds.

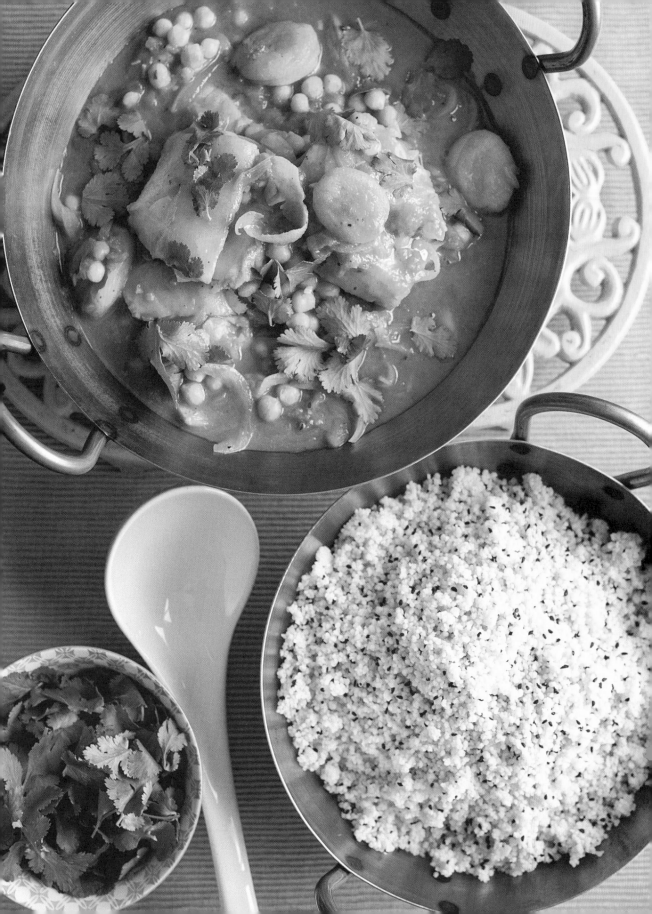

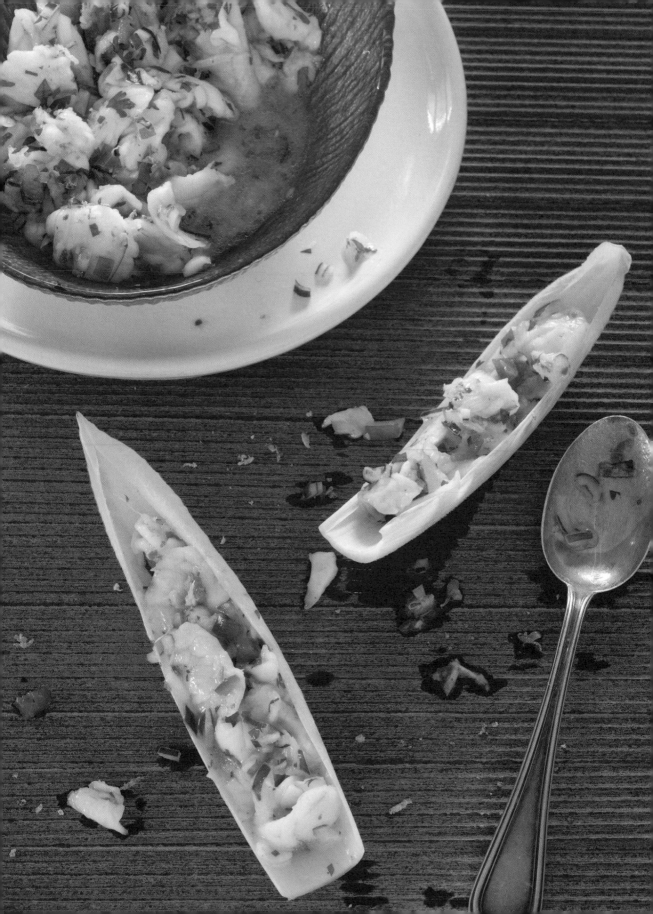

SEA BASS CEVICHE WITH CHICORY

Tangy, fresh and light, this Peruvian classic takes very little time to prepare; the effort you have to put into some careful chopping is amply rewarded by the vibrant result. Find the freshest possible sea bass, ideally from a fishmonger, and ask for it to be filleted, with any pin bones removed.

READY IN **20** MINUTES

To make the marinade, combine the lime juice, soy sauce and sugar in a small bowl and whisk to dissolve the sugar.

Next, use a very sharp knife to slice the sea bass; place each fillet on a board with the tail end on your right. Holding the knife at a shallow angle, slice the flesh almost horizontally toward the tail, stopping before you slice through the skin. This should give you very thin slices of fish (like slices of smoked salmon).

Place the sliced sea bass into a shallow dish along with the onion, chilli and coriander/cilantro. Pour over the marinade and stir gently to coat the fish. Cover and leave to marinate for 10 minutes, stirring once or twice during this time.

Slice the ends from the chicory/Belgian endive and tear off the leaves, keeping them whole. Serve the ceviche with the chicory/Belgian endive leaves, with the olive oil drizzled over the ceviche. Let everyone help themselves, scooping the sea bass into the large leaves to serve.

SERVES 4

juice of 6 limes

3 tbsp soy sauce

½ tsp sugar

4 sea bass fillets

1 red onion, finely chopped

1 red chilli, deseeded and finely chopped

handful of coriander/cilantro leaves, chopped

2 chicory/Belgian endive heads

1 tbsp olive oil

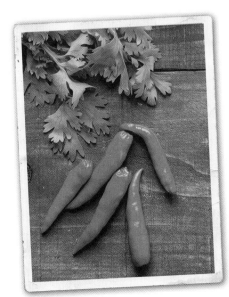

SEA BASS WITH THAI VEGETABLES

Light and healthy, this recipe is full of vibrant Thai flavours that make it satisfying without being laden with carbs or calories. If you're particularly hungry, rice noodles go very well with this dish and once cooked can be tossed through the vegetable noodles. I use a julienne peeler to quickly shred the vegetables into thin strips but you could also use a spiralizer or, if you're completely without tools, just shred the vegetables into the finest strips you can manage using a sharp knife.

SERVES 4

READY IN **20** MINUTES

sesame or rapeseed/canola oil, for cooking

4 carrots, peeled and julienned

¼ savoy cabbage, finely shredded

2 red peppers, deseeded and julienned

4 courgettes/zucchini, julienned

2 garlic cloves, grated

1 green chilli, deseeded and finely chopped

2cm/¾in piece of root ginger, peeled and grated

small handful coriander/cilantro leaves, roughly chopped

2 tbsp fish sauce

4 tbsp soy sauce

2 tbsp sesame seeds, toasted

4 sea bass fillets

juice of 1 lime

sea salt and freshly ground black pepper

Heat 2 tablespoons of the oil in a large frying pan or wok until almost smoking hot. Add the carrots, cabbage and most of the red peppers and stir fry for 3–4 minutes until just softened. Then throw in the courgettes/zucchini, garlic, chilli and ginger and cook for a further 3–4 minutes, tossing and stirring frequently.

Add most of the coriander/cilantro, the fish sauce and soy sauce and cook for 1 minute to flavour the vegetables with the seasoning. Stir through the sesame seeds and leave to one side while you cook the fish.

Score the skin-side of the sea bass with a sharp knife, then season with salt and pepper on both sides. Heat a little more oil in a frying pan and place the fish into the pan skin-side down; the oil should sizzle when the fish goes in. Cook for 2–3 minutes until the edges are just crispy, flip over, squeeze in the lime juice and cook for 2 minutes until the fish is cooked through.

Serve each fillet of sea bass on top of a pile of the stir-fried vegetables, sprinkled with the remaining coriander/cilantro. Finely chop the remaining red pepper and sprinkle over.

NOTE: If you decide to use rice noodles, cook them according to the package directions while you are cooking the vegetables and then add to the stir-fried vegetables along with the fish and soy sauces.

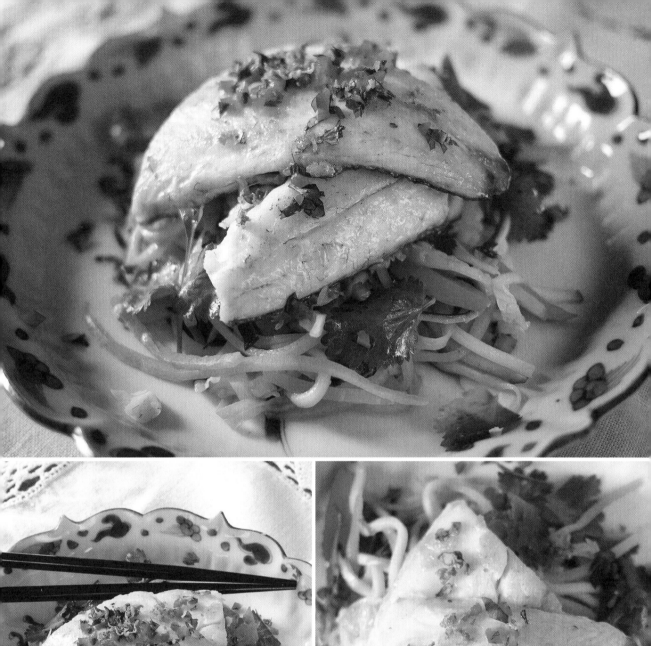
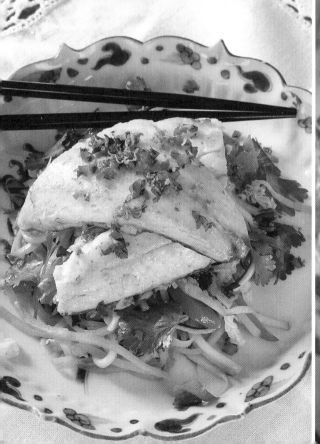
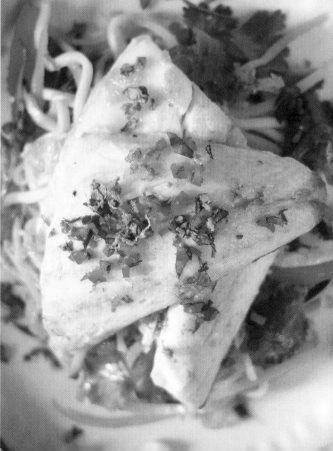

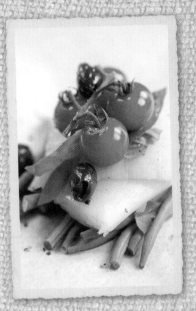

COD, GREEN BEAN AND CHERRY TOMATO PARCELS

Baked in a parcel, this delicate fish retains all of its moisture while taking on plenty of flavour from the other ingredients. Serve with tender new, salad potatoes which will soak up all of the cooking juices when crushed with the back of your fork.

READY IN 20 MINUTES

SERVES 4

200g/7oz fine/French beans

4 cod fillets (each about 120–140g/ 4–5 oz)

4 small bunches of cherry tomatoes (each with about 5–6 tomatoes)

2 tbsp pitted black olives

olive oil, for drizzling

½ lemon

1 tbsp pine nuts

16 basil leaves

200ml/7fl oz/¾ cup white wine

sea salt and freshly ground black pepper

Preheat the oven to 190°C/375°F/gas 5.

Cut four pieces of baking parchment large enough to form a parcel for each piece of cod.

Place the green beans in equal piles in the middle of each piece of paper. Lay the cod fillets on top of each pile, followed by a bunch of cherry tomatoes and a few olives. Drizzle each with a little olive oil, followed by a squeeze of lemon juice and a few pine nuts. Tear each basil leaf in half before placing them on top. Season with salt and pepper.

Partially seal the parcels by twisting the edges of the paper together at both ends so that when you add the white wine it won't leak out. Pour the wine into the parcels, then finish sealing the edges and top of the parcels and place them on a baking sheet.

Bake in the middle of the oven for 15 minutes until the fish is cooked through and the vegetables are tender. When you're ready to serve, lift the whole parcels onto the plates, open the edges and dive in.

BAKED SMOKED HADDOCK WITH ROASTED CELERIAC

Earthy, aniseedy celeriac complements the smoked haddock and ham in this quick one-dish recipe. Celeriac's woody texture means that once cut into wedges it crisps easily in the oven, giving plenty of bite and flavour. A dollop of Grainy Mustard Mayonnaise (see page 169) served on top and a green salad finishes the dish perfectly.

Preheat the oven to 200°C/400°F/gas 6.

Place the celeriac and potato wedges in a bowl with the mustard and nigella seeds. Add the oil, some salt and pepper and toss together well. Spread out on a baking sheet and roast on the top shelf for 25 minutes, removing the sheet halfway through and tossing the vegetables to help them cook evenly.

Meanwhile, wrap each piece of haddock in a slice of Parma ham/prosciutto and if you're making your own mayonnaise, now's the time to do that.

After the 25 minutes is up, take the celeriac and potatoes out of the oven, place the ham-wrapped fish fillets on top and return to the middle of the oven for 10 minutes until the fish is cooked through.

Remove from the oven and squeeze the lemon over the top of the fish and scatter with parsley. Serve with green salad and the Grainy Mustard Mayonnaise.

READY IN 40 MINUTES

SERVES 4

1 celeriac (about 750g/1lb 10oz) peeled and cut into wedges

2 large white potatoes (about 400g/14oz), peeled and cut into wedges

1 tsp yellow mustard seeds

1 tsp nigella (black onion) seeds

1–2 tbsp rapeseed/canola oil

4 smoked haddock fillets (each about 170g/6oz)

4 slices Parma ham/prosciutto

juice of ½ lemon

handful of parsley, roughly chopped

sea salt and freshly ground black pepper

green salad, to serve

Grainy Mustard Mayonnaise (see page 169), to serve

NOTE: Mashed celeriac is also a delicious accompaniment to other smoked fish or game in the autumn. I like it cooked in salted water until soft and then roughly mashed with butter and seasoning, so that there's still plenty of texture.

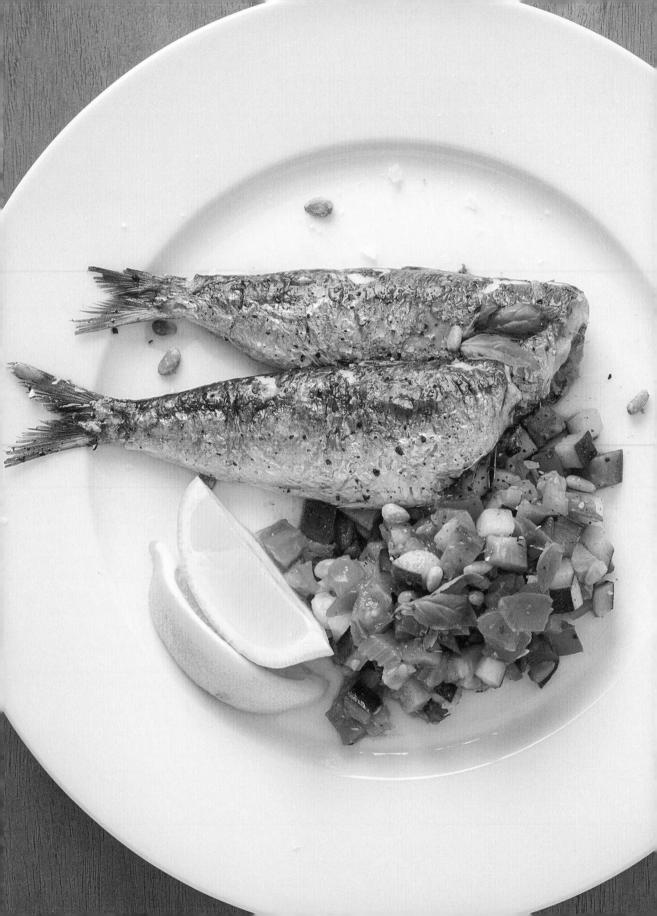

GRILLED SARDINES WITH WARM CAPONATA

This quick version of the classic Sicilian vegetable stew, caponata, is a delicious accompaniment to oily fish like sardines and mackerel. Best served slightly warm or cold, it is similar to ratatouille, being even better on day two when the flavours have had a little time to develop.

Heat a generous slug of olive oil in a wide frying pan over a medium heat and cook the celery and onion for 5 minutes until softened.

Add the aubergine/eggplant, courgettes/zucchini and garlic, cover with a lid and cook for 10 minutes; check halfway through and add more olive oil if the mixture looks too dry. Stir in the tomato purée/paste, chopped tomatoes and parsley and bring to a simmer. Cook for another 10 minutes, stirring often before seasoning with a pinch of sugar, salt and pepper.

Meanwhile, heat a non-stick frying pan and add the pine nuts. Stir for 2–3 minutes until they start to colour, then remove and leave to one side.

Add the capers, pine nuts and the vinegar and leave the caponata to rest in the pan while you grill/broil the sardines.

Preheat the grill/broiler to high. Rub the sardines with a little olive oil, salt and pepper and place on a foil-lined sheet. Grill for about 4 minutes on each side until the skin has started to blister and blacken and the fish is cooked through.

Carefully lift the sardines onto plates and serve with a pile of caponata and wedges of lemon and tear the basil leaves over the top.

NOTE: I love olives, especially the piquant Italian green ones; try adding these to the caponata if you're a fan, or perhaps experiment by adding a finely chopped red chilli or juicy sultanas/golden raisins.

READY IN 40 MINUTES

SERVES 4

olive oil, for cooking

½ celery stalk, finely chopped

1 red onion, chopped

1 small aubergine/eggplant, diced into 5mm/¼in cubes

2 small courgettes/zucchini, diced into 5mm/¼in cubes

1 garlic clove, finely chopped

1 heaped tsp tomato purée/paste

4 tomatoes, diced

handful of parsley, chopped

pinch of brown sugar

1 tbsp pine nuts

1 tbsp capers

splash of red wine vinegar

8 sardines (the freshest you can find)

sea salt and freshly ground black pepper

1 lemon, cut into wedges, to serve

handful of basil leaves, to serve

GARLIC ROAST SALMON WITH COURGETTES AND OLIVES

Lightly roasting courgettes/zucchini with garlic and herbs brings out their sweet flavour without losing their naturally sweet crunch. I use a mixture of yellow and green courgettes/zucchini in this recipe but do just use green if the yellow ones prove elusive.

SERVES 4

READY IN 30 MINUTES

3 large courgettes/zucchini

3 garlic cloves, sliced

2 tbsp olive oil

16 cherry tomatoes

4 salmon fillets

2 lemon wedges

handful of parsley, chopped

handful of basil, chopped

16 pitted black olives

sea salt and freshly ground black pepper

Preheat the oven to 190°C/375°F/gas 5.

Slice the courgettes/zucchini diagonally into bite-size chunks. Place in a bowl with the garlic, olive oil and some salt and pepper and toss together. Line a deep roasting tray with baking paper. Spread out the coated courgettes/zucchini, scatter over the cherry tomatoes and place the salmon on top of the vegetables.

Squeeze the juice from the lemon wedges over the salmon and then nestle the wedges among the vegetables. Sprinkle over the parsley. Place in the middle of the oven and bake for 15 minutes until the fish is cooked through.

Take the tray out of the oven, lift off the salmon fillets and leave to one side on a warm plate. Add the basil and olives to the tray and stir to mix through the courgette/zucchini mixture. Return the tray to the oven for 5 minutes until everything is warmed through.

Serve the salmon on top of the vegetable and olive mixture.

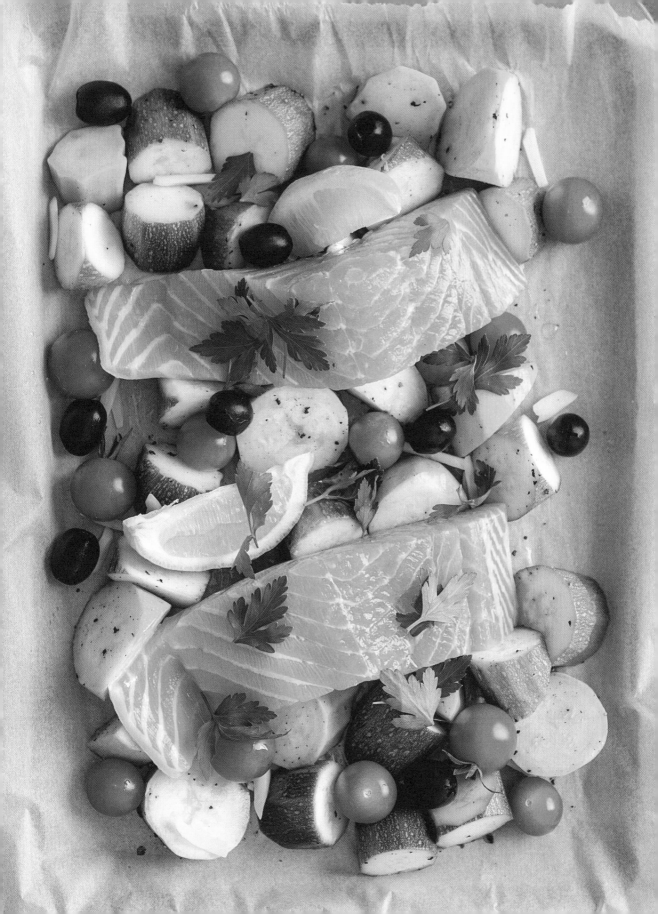

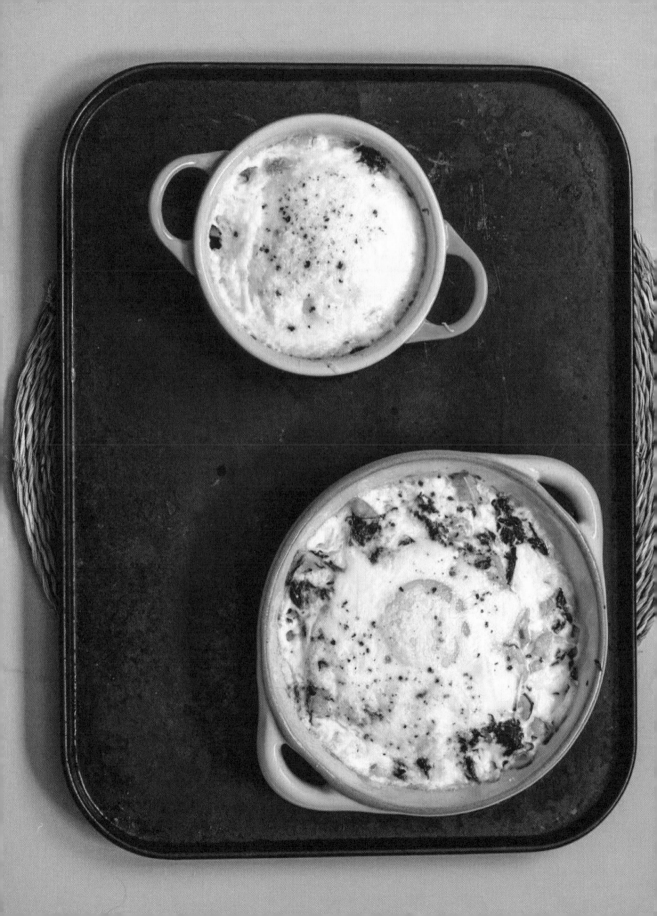

BAKED EGGS WITH SALMON AND SPINACH

Rich and satisfying, this egg dish feels like something really indulgent. You will need four small, shallow baking dishes, or failing that, four large ramekins. Lovely served with toast.

Preheat the oven to 180°C/350°F/gas 4.

Lightly butter four baking dishes or ramekins.

Rinse the spinach under cool running water and then place in a large saucepan. Cook for 1–2 minutes until the leaves have wilted. Drain, then squeeze out as much liquid as you can.

Roughly chop the spinach on a board and place in a bowl with the salmon. Season with salt and pepper and add a drizzle of olive oil and the lemon juice. Mix gently.

Divide the mixture between the four dishes or ramekins, pressing down lightly. Make a slight well in the middle of each dish and crack the eggs into the centres, with the yolk in the middle. Spoon the double/heavy cream on top, season with black pepper and then grate over a little Parmesan.

Place the dishes on a baking sheet and bake in the middle of the oven for 15 minutes until the whites of the eggs have set and the Parmesan has turned slightly golden; the yolks should still have a bit of a wobble.

READY IN 20 MINUTES

SERVES 4

butter, for greasing
200g/7oz/4 cups spinach leaves
200g/7oz smoked salmon, sliced
olive oil, for drizzling
squeeze of lemon juice
4 large eggs
4 tbsp double/heavy cream
Parmesan cheese, for grating
sea salt and freshly ground black pepper

NOTE: If you don't have four individual dishes, you could make the entire recipe in one large ovenproof dish.

LIME AND CORIANDER CRUSTED TUNA WITH BEAN SALSA

The lime crust in this recipe is a delicious contrast to the soft, rare tuna. Choose tuna that is as fresh as possible. It takes no time to throw together the refreshing bean salsa, which is almost a meal in itself. If you can't find a ripe avocado for the salsa, substitute sweetcorn kernels instead.

SERVES 4

READY IN **15** MINUTES

4 tsp black peppercorns

4 tsp coriander seeds

2 tsp salt

zest of 3 limes

4 tuna steaks (each about 125g/4½oz)

rapeseed/canola oil, for frying

lime wedges, to serve

FOR THE SALSA

400g/14oz canned black-eyed, aduki or mixed beans, drained

4 tomatoes, deseeded and diced

1 avocado, peeled, pitted and diced

½ red onion, finely chopped

1 garlic clove, finely chopped

1 red chilli, finely chopped

2 tbsp olive oil

juice of 3 limes

handful of coriander/cilantro leaves, roughly chopped

sea salt and freshly ground black pepper

Using a pestle and mortar, if you have one, crush the peppercorns and coriander seeds. If you don't have one, use the end of a rolling pin to crush them in a small bowl. Mix the salt and lime zest into the crushed seeds and tip out onto a large flat plate.

Firmly press the tuna steaks into the seed mixture, turning them over to coat evenly on both sides. Leave to one side.

To make the salsa, tip the beans into a bowl and add the tomatoes, avocado, onion, garlic and chilli. Add the olive oil, half of the lime juice, the coriander/cilantro and a little salt and pepper. Mix well.

Heat a little oil in a frying pan and when hot, add the tuna steaks. Sear for 1 minute on each side, or more if you prefer tuna well cooked. Remove from the pan, slice in half diagonally and serve with the bean salsa and wedges of lime to squeeze over.

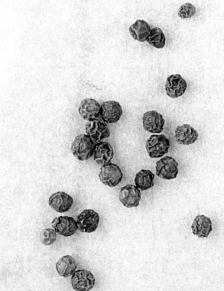

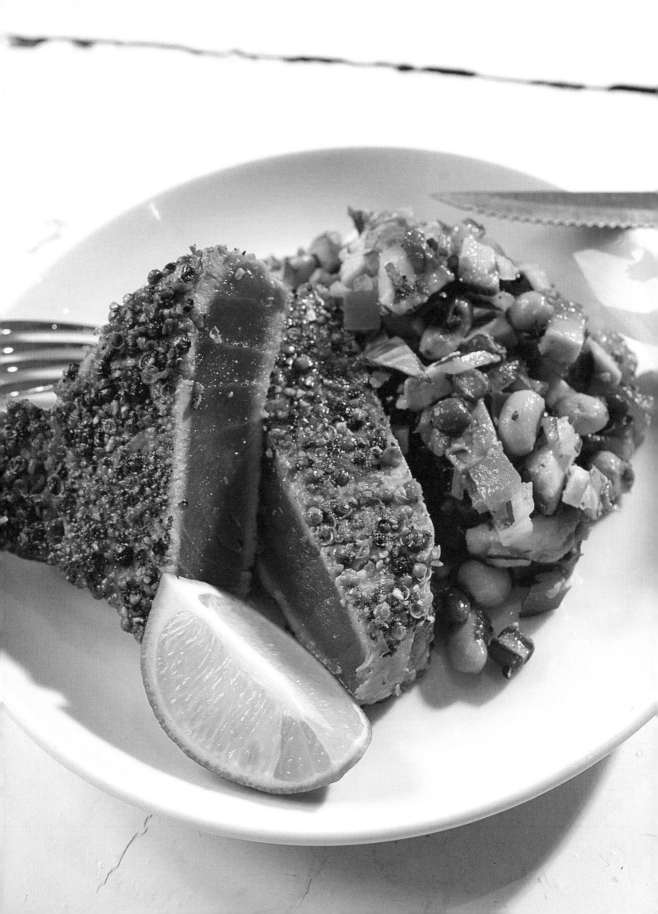

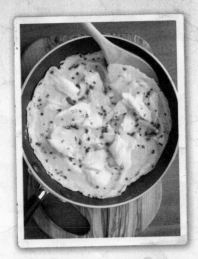

SMOKED HADDOCK, CHIVE AND GRUYÈRE OMELETTE

Flakes of smoked haddock, fluffy beaten eggs and garden chives make a light supper that is ready in a matter of minutes. This is a lighter version of the classic Omelette Arnold Bennett without the heaviness or extra work of a béchamel sauce. You can either make one large omelette as below, or divide the mixture into four and make individual omelettes.

READY IN 20 MINUTES

SERVES 4

250g/9oz smoked haddock fillets

olive oil, for cooking

55g/2oz Gruyère cheese

10 large eggs

4 tbsp crème fraîche

small bunch of chives, finely chopped

55g/2oz/¼ cup butter

freshly ground black pepper

handful of watercress or spinach, to serve

NOTE: Smoked salmon in place of the haddock is also delicious and is even quicker as it doesn't need any pre-cooking. Roughly chop the salmon and flake into the omelette as above.

Preheat the oven to 180°C/350°F/gas 4.

Place the haddock fillets on a large piece of foil, drizzle over a little olive oil, grind over some pepper and seal the edges of the foil to create an airtight parcel. Place on a baking sheet in the middle of the oven for 10–15 minutes until just cooked through. Lift the fish out of the foil parcel and once slightly cooled, flake into small pieces, discarding any skin or bones.

Meanwhile, grate or peel the Gruyère into shavings and leave to one side. Whisk together the eggs and crème fraîche with a little pepper (the fish is so salty you won't need any additional salt) and stir in half of the chives.

Melt the butter in a large frying pan over a medium-high heat until sizzling and beginning to turn golden. Test the pan is hot enough by pouring in a drizzle of egg to check that it immediately sizzles and sets.

Quickly pour all of the egg mixture into the pan and scatter the flaked haddock over the top. Use a wooden spoon or spatula to draw the set edges of the omelette into the middle of the pan as it cooks, allowing the still raw egg mix to flood to the edges of the pan.

Scatter over the remaining chives and the Gruyère and cook for 1–2 minutes until the egg has nearly set; there should still be a bit of a wobble.

Fold the omelette in half as you slide it out of the pan onto a plate and serve cut into slices with a salad of watercress and spinach leaves.

PRAWN, GREEN CHILLI AND TOMATO CURRY

The natural sweetness of the shallots and prawns/shrimp in this recipe is balanced by the sharp tomatoes and lime. Buy the best fresh tomatoes you can get your hands on and only use one of the green chillies if you prefer a milder curry.

Heat the oil in a large frying pan. Add the shallots and fry for 5 minutes until softened. Add the ginger, garlic and chillies and cook for another 5 minutes. Add the ground coriander and turmeric, mustard seeds and tomato purée/paste and stir well, frying for 1 minute.

Add the tomatoes and stock. Bring to the boil, then turn down the heat and simmer for 10 minutes, stirring occasionally. Taste and add a little salt and pepper and a pinch of sugar if the sauce is sharp.

Tip in the prawns/shrimp, bring back to a simmer and cook for 3–5 minutes until the prawns are cooked through, adding a little more stock if there isn't enough liquid in the pan. Remove the pan from the heat and stir in the crème fraîche, lime juice and coriander/cilantro.

Serve with rice and some sweet chutney, if you like.

READY IN 30 MINUTES

SERVES 4

2 tbsp rapeseed/canola oil

4 banana shallots, sliced

2cm/¾in piece of root ginger, peeled and grated

2 garlic cloves, finely chopped

1–2 green chillies, deseeded and finely chopped

1 tsp ground coriander

½ tsp ground turmeric

1 tsp yellow mustard seeds

1 tsp tomato purée/paste

8 large tomatoes, chopped

350ml/12fl oz/1½ cups fish or vegetable stock

brown sugar, to taste (optional)

500g/1lb 2oz raw king prawns/jumbo shrimp

2 tbsp crème fraîche

juice of 1 lime

handful of coriander/cilantro leaves, roughly chopped

sea salt and freshly ground black pepper

steamed rice and sweet chutney, to serve (optional)

NOTE: You could use a firm-fleshed fish in place of the prawns such as haddock, pollock or monkfish if you like.

SPICY PRAWN AND TOMATO SPAGHETTI

READY IN 20 MINUTES

SERVES 4

2 tbsp rapeseed/canola oil

1 garlic clove, chopped

1 red chilli, deseeded and finely chopped

6 tomatoes, chopped

1 heaped tsp tomato purée/paste

2 heaped tbsp crème fraîche

2 handfuls of parsley, chopped

squeeze of lemon juice

400g/14oz small cooked, peeled prawns/shrimp

pinch of brown sugar, to taste (optional)

340g/12oz spaghetti

2–3 tbsp olive oil

sea salt and freshly ground black pepper

NOTE: You can use raw prawns/shrimp for this recipe too. Add them to the pan when you stir in the crème fraîche and then follow the recipe as normal.

A light and summery pasta dish ideal to eat in the evening sunshine with a cold glass of white wine. You can make it your own by adding olives, capers or perhaps some sliced, sun-dried tomatoes. Serve with a peppery spinach and Parmesan salad.

Heat the rapeseed/canola oil in a pan that will later be large enough to take the cooked spaghetti. When hot, add the garlic and chilli and cook for about 2 minutes until softened. Add the tomatoes and cook for 5 minutes, stirring occasionally.

Stir in the tomato purée/paste, crème fraîche and most of the parsley along with the lemon juice and a sprinkling of salt and pepper. Bring to a simmer and cook for 3–4 minutes to allow the sauce to thicken. Tip in the prawns/shrimp, bring back to a simmer to heat through and then taste the sauce. If the tomatoes are quite acidic you may need to add a pinch of sugar.

Meanwhile, bring a pan of salted water to the boil. Add the spaghetti and cook for about 8–10 minutes until just al dente (cooked, but still with a little bite) before draining and tossing through the olive oil.

Return the tomato and prawn mixture to a medium heat. Add the spaghetti and toss really well using a pair of tongs, to give the pasta a chance to absorb some of the sauce.

Pile onto serving plates or take to the table as it is and scatter over the remaining parsley.

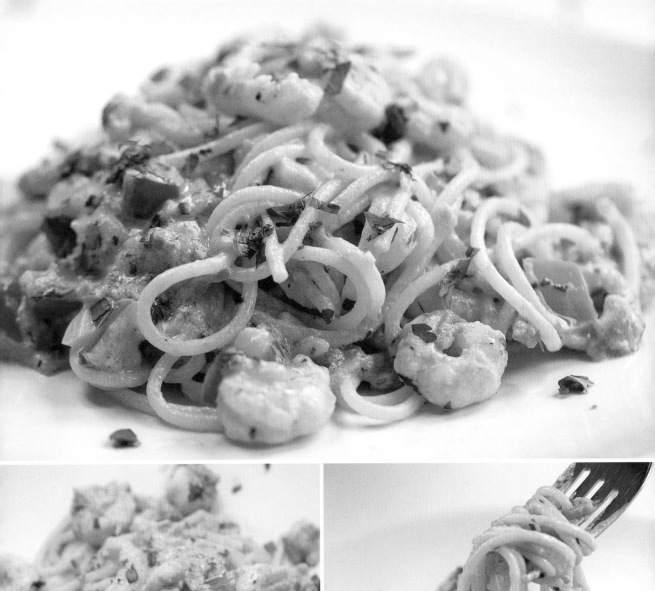

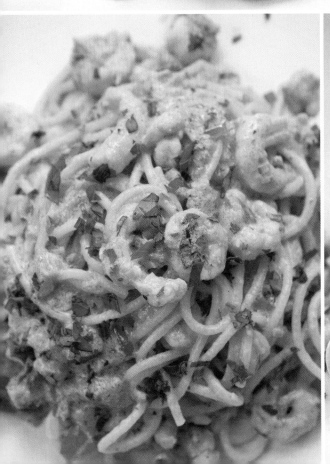

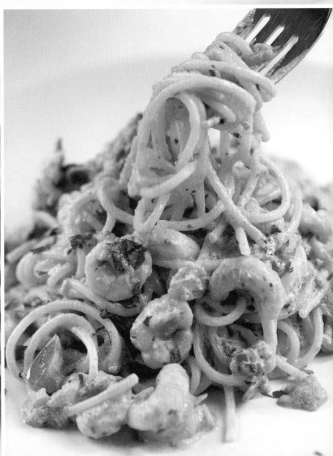

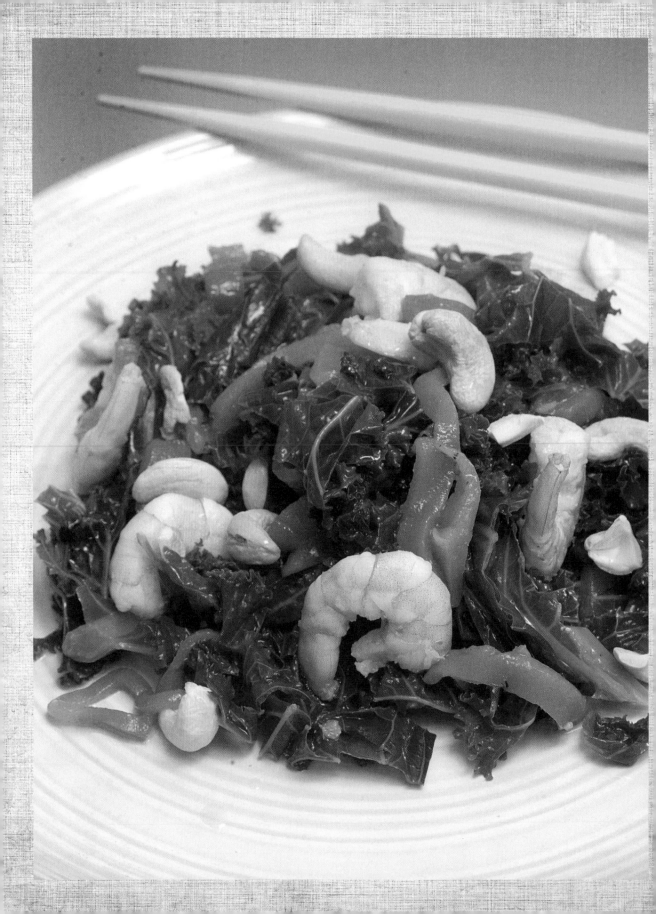

CURLY KALE, KING PRAWN AND CASHEW STIR-FRY

Earthy, minerally and packed with nutrients, curly kale has a pleasant bitterness that works well with salty, smoky flavours, such as bacon or blue cheese. In this recipe, stir-fried with Asian flavours, kale makes a welcome stand-in for pak choi/bok choy or cabbage. Try serving this stir-fry with steamed rice or rice noodles.

READY IN
15
MINUTES

Preheat the oven to 200°C/400°F/gas 6.

Spread the cashews on a baking sheet and bake in the middle of the oven for 8–10 minutes until golden.

Meanwhile, bring a pan of salted water to the boil. Shred the kale into thin ribbons (if it isn't pre-chopped already) and cook it in the boiling water for 2 minutes. Drain, rinse under cold running water, then leave to one side.

Mix the lime juice, soy sauce and fish sauce together in a small bowl with the sugar, stirring to dissolve the sugar.

Heat the oil in a large pan or wok until almost smoking and add the garlic and chilli. Fry for 2 minutes before adding the ginger and prawns/shrimp and continue to fry until the prawns/shrimp have just turned opaque.

Add the red peppers and blanched kale and toss everything together over the heat for another 2 minutes or so, adding more oil if needed.

Pour over the lime, soy sauce and fish sauce mixture, stir well and cook for a further 1–2 minutes to reduce the sauce. Toss the roasted cashew nuts through the stir-fry and serve.

SERVES 4

2 tbsp cashew nuts

300g/10½oz curly kale

juice of 1 lime

3 tbsp soy sauce

1 tbsp fish sauce

pinch of brown sugar

2 tbsp rapeseed/canola oil, plus extra if needed

2 garlic cloves, sliced

1 red chilli, deseeded and sliced

2cm/¾in piece of root ginger, peeled and grated

300g/10½oz raw peeled king prawns/jumbo shrimp

2 roasted red peppers (available in jars), sliced

WARM SQUID AND COURGETTE SALAD WITH CHORIZO AND MINT

Fresh squid is widely available and compared to other fish is inexpensive. Ask your fishmonger to prepare the squid for you, removing the beak and membrane but keeping the tentacles, which are delicious. If you don't have a griddle/grill pan, you can cook the squid in a large frying pan instead. When they're in season, use yellow courgettes/zucchini if you can find them as they look great in this salad.

SERVES 4

READY IN **20** *MINUTES*

55g/2oz/½ cup pine nuts

3 courgettes/zucchini

85g/3oz/2½ cups rocket/arugula

10 mint leaves, roughly chopped

115g/4oz cooking chorizo, sliced diagonally

2 whole squid, cleaned

1 garlic clove, finely sliced

juice of ½ lemon

8 sun-dried tomatoes, sliced

sea salt and freshly ground black pepper

extra virgin olive oil, for drizzling

55g/2oz Parmesan cheese, for grating

Preheat the oven to 190°C/375°F/gas 5.

Spread the pine nuts on a baking sheet and roast in the middle of the oven for 8–10 minutes until golden.

Meanwhile, cut the courgettes/zucchini into wide ribbons using a potato peeler. Place the courgettes/zucchini in a large salad bowl with the rocket/arugula and mint. Leave to one side.

Heat a griddle/grill pan or frying pan and once hot add the chorizo. Cook for 4–5 minutes, turning halfway through, until the chorizo caramelizes slightly at the edges and releases plenty of oil. Remove from the pan with a slotted spoon, leaving the oil in the pan.

Slice the squid in half and then into fat strips, keeping the strips quite large as they will curl up and shrink when you cook them. Return the chorizo pan to the heat and when sizzling, add the squid and garlic. Season with salt and pepper and cook for 2–3 minutes, tossing every so often. Add the lemon juice and sun-dried tomatoes, remove from the heat and stir well.

Tip the squid onto the courgette/zucchini salad followed by a drizzle of olive oil and the roasted pine nuts. Grate over the Parmesan, in large flakes. Taste the salad to check if it needs more salt of pepper or another squeeze of lemon juice. Toss together well and then serve with a little more Parmesan flaked on top.

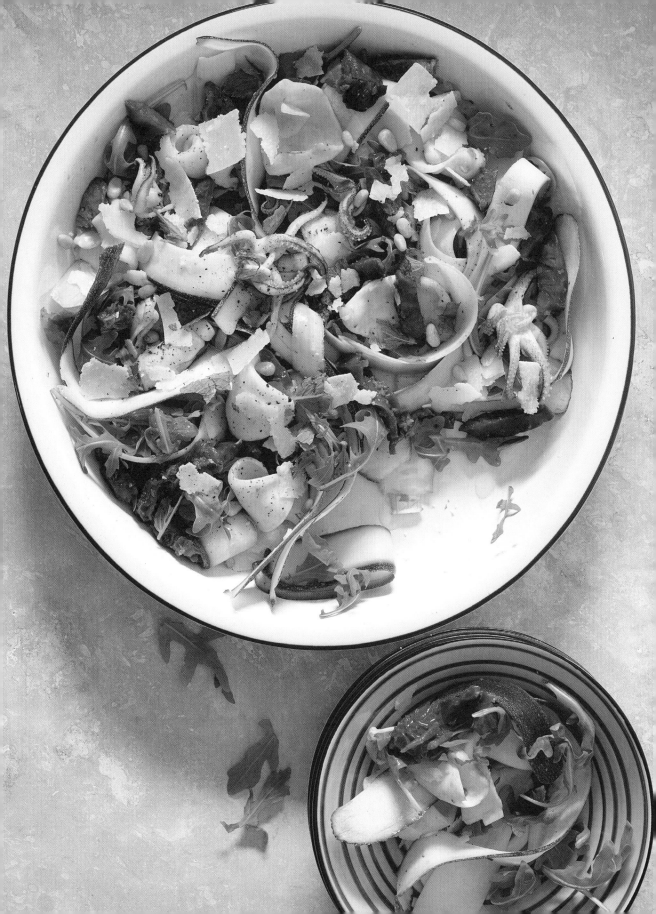

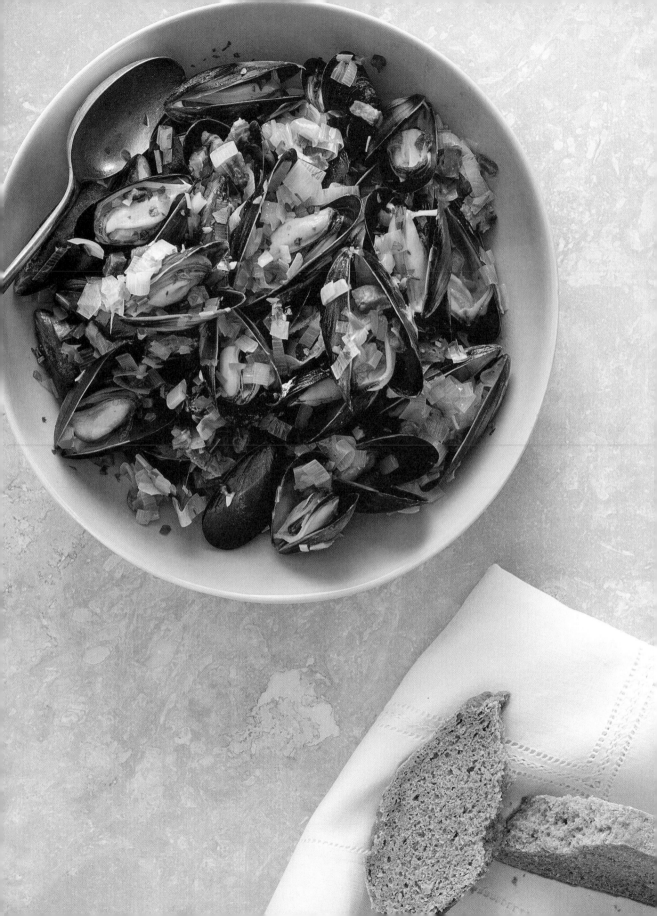

MUSSELS WITH LEEKS AND CHORIZO

Packed with smoky flavour, this combination of Spanish sausage and shellfish is a classic pairing. It's comforting, satiating and painless to prepare. Most fishmongers now sell mussels already cleaned, saving you a lot of time scraping and de-bearding.

Start off by cleaning the mussels: thoroughly scrub the mussels under cold running water and rinse well. Remove any beards by pulling them toward the large part of the shell. If any of the mussels are open, tap them hard against a work surface and if they don't close, discard them.

Heat a deep saucepan (large enough to take all of the mussels) over a medium heat and add the chorizo. You won't need any additional oil in the pan because the chorizo releases so much of its own during cooking. Fry for about 5 minutes, stirring every so often, until it changes colour to a deep, caramelized red.

Add the leek, garlic and chilli to the pan and cook for a further 5 minutes before stirring in the tomato purée/paste. Pour the white wine into the pan, season with salt and pepper and then tip in the mussels.

Bring to the boil, cover the pan with a lid and cook for 3–4 minutes or until the shells have opened.

Spoon the mussels and plenty of the cooking liquor into serving bowls, discarding any that haven't opened. Scatter over the parsley and serve with plenty of crusty bread.

SERVES 4

READY IN 20 MINUTES

2kg/4lb 8oz fresh mussels (in their shells)

170g/6oz cooking chorizo, diced

1 large leek, finely sliced

2 garlic cloves, sliced

1 red chilli, deseeded and finely chopped

1 heaped tsp tomato purée/paste

400ml/14fl oz/1¾ cups white wine

sea salt and freshly ground black pepper

handful of parsley, roughly chopped

crusty bread, to serve

NOTE: This recipe works really well with smoked bacon lardons in place of the chorizo or with cider in place of the white wine.

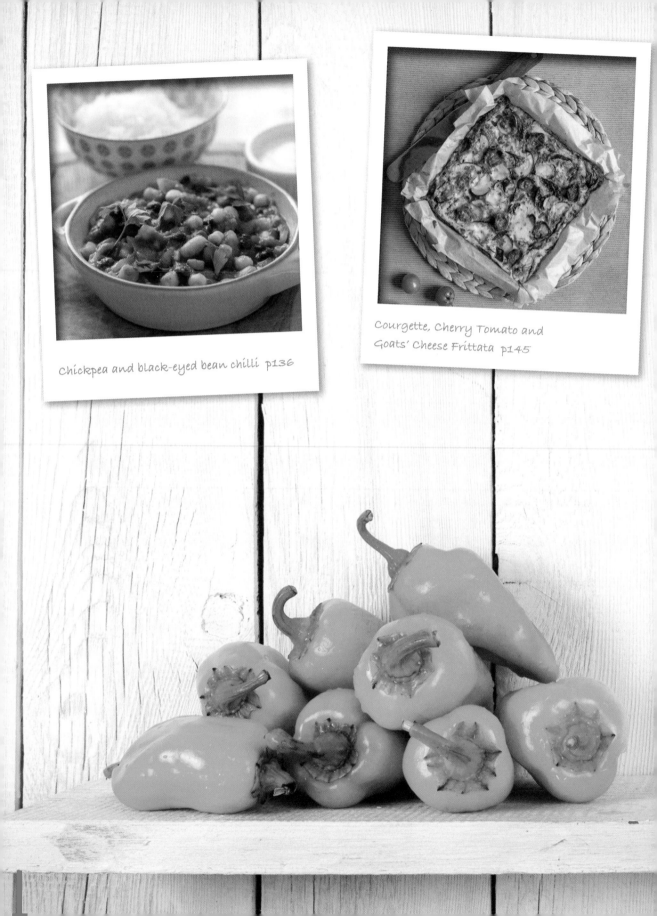

Chickpea and black-eyed bean chilli p136

Courgette, Cherry Tomato and Goats' Cheese Frittata p145

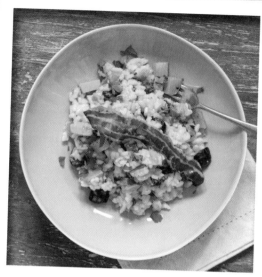

Butternut squash, chestnut and sage risotto p150

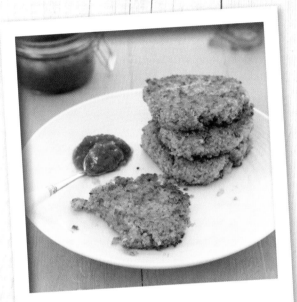

Quinoa, courgette and herb cakes p160

GRAINS, PULSES & VEGETABLES

AUBERGINE, SPINACH AND RED LENTIL CURRY

Full of spices, this mellow curry is a great example of how satisfying vegetarian cooking can be. Served with a few chapatti or naan breads and chutney, it's quite delicious and, without meat, it's great value, too.

SERVES 4

READY IN 40 MINUTES

rapeseed/canola oil, for cooking

6 baby or 2 large aubergines/eggplants, sliced into wedges

1 onion, sliced

1 green chilli, deseeded and finely chopped

2cm/¾in piece of root ginger, peeled and grated

2 garlic cloves, finely chopped

1 tsp yellow mustard seeds

2 tsp garam masala

1 tsp tomato purée/paste

6 tomatoes, roughly diced

115g/4oz/¾ cup dried red lentils

300ml/10½fl oz/1¼ cups vegetable stock

225g/8oz/4½ cups spinach leaves

400ml/14fl oz/1¾ cups coconut milk

sea salt and freshly ground black pepper

handful of coriander/cilantro leaves, roughly chopped, for sprinkling

plain yogurt and nigella (black onion) seeds, to serve (optional)

Heat 2 tablespoons of oil in a large frying pan and cook the aubergine/eggplant wedges in batches on both sides for about 5 minutes until browned. Remove from the pan and leave to one side.

Add the onion with a little more oil and cook for 5 minutes before adding the chilli, ginger and garlic. Cook for another 5 minutes until the onion has softened. Add the mustard seeds, garam masala and tomato purée/paste and stir until the mustard seeds begin to make a popping sound.

Add the tomatoes to the pan along with the red lentils and stock. Add a pinch of salt, stir and bring to a gentle simmer. Cook for 10 minutes, stirring occasionally to stop the vegetables sticking to the bottom of the pan and adding a little more stock if the curry looks too dry.

Meanwhile, bring a large pan of salted water to the boil and add the spinach. Cook for 1–2 minutes until wilted. Drain, then squeeze out as much liquid from the leaves as you can.

Pour the coconut milk into the curry, stir well and then add the cooked aubergines along with the drained spinach. Bring back to a gentle simmer and leave to bubble for 2–3 minutes until the curry is piping hot. Serve scattered with the coriander/cilantro and with plain yogurt sprinkled with a few nigella seeds, if you like.

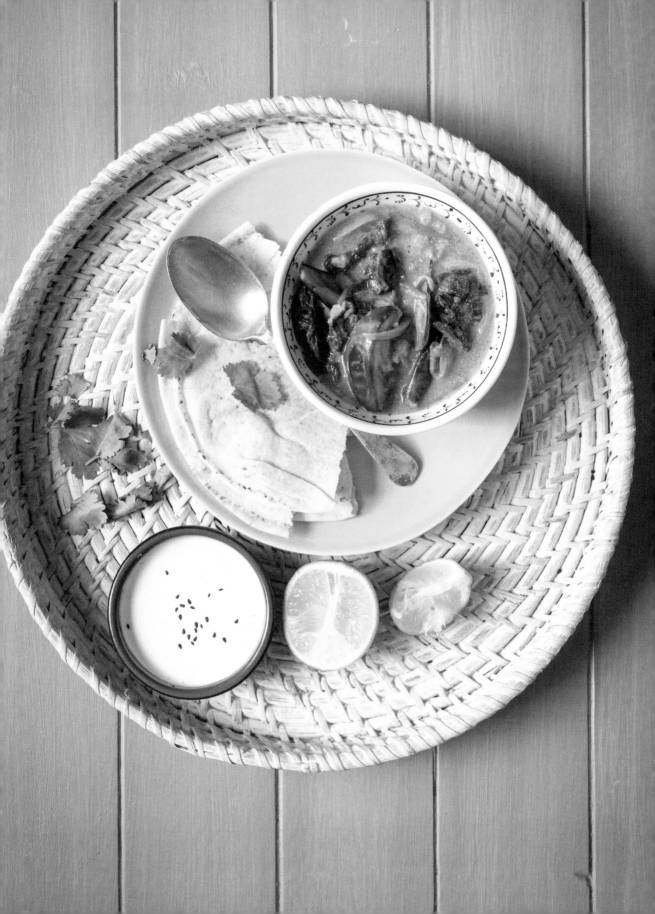

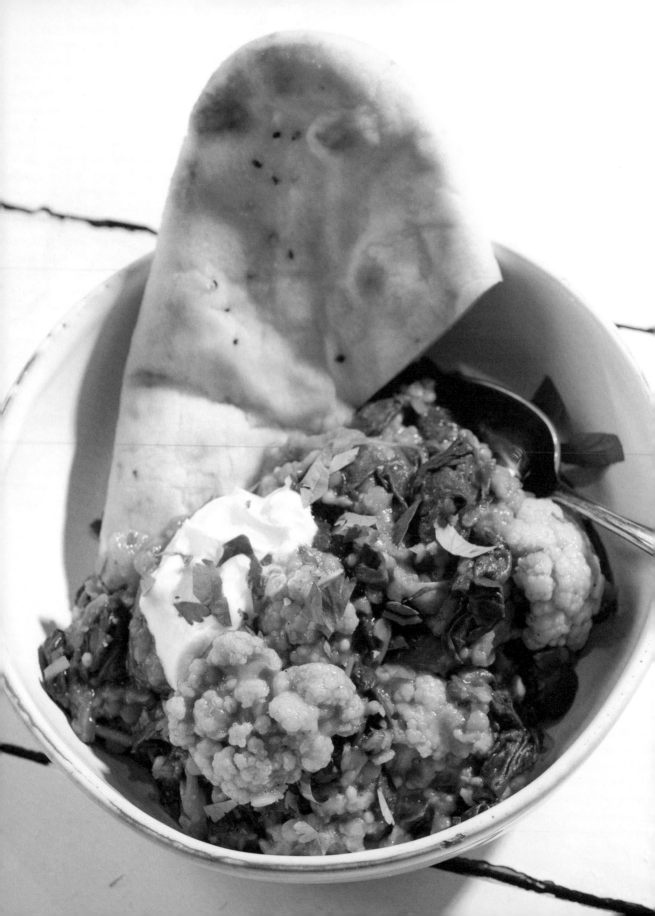

SPINACH AND CAULIFLOWER DHAL

This is a fragrant one-pot supper full of nutritious ingredients and brought to life by warming, mild, Indian spices. This could also be served as the vegetable accompaniment to a main course.

Heat a generous slug of oil over a medium heat in a large casserole pan and add the onion. Cook for 5 minutes, then add the garlic and chilli and continue to cook until softened and translucent.

Add the tomato purée/paste, mustard seeds, garam masala and turmeric and cook for 2 minutes, stirring to stop the onion and spices sticking to the bottom of the pan. If it seems very dry, add a little more oil. Add the lentils, stirring over the heat for 1 minute.

Pour in half of the stock, bring to the boil, then reduce the heat and simmer for 5 minutes, covered with a lid. Add the cauliflower and another 300ml/10½fl oz/1¼ cups of the stock along with plenty of salt and pepper. Cover with a lid and simmer for 15 minutes.

Meanwhile, wash the spinach and place in a large pan over a medium-high heat. Cover with a lid and cook for 2–3 minutes until the leaves have wilted. Drain, then squeeze out as much moisture as you can.

Keep stirring and checking the lentils and cauliflower, adding more stock if needed to stop the mixture drying out. When the cauliflower is tender and the lentils completely cooked, stir in the spinach and lemon juice and then taste to check the seasoning. Leave to stand for a few minutes, then scatter with chopped coriander/cilantro. Serve with yogurt and naan bread, if you like.

READY IN 40 MINUTES

SERVES 4

rapeseed/canola oil, for frying

1 onion, finely sliced

2 garlic cloves, crushed

1 green chilli, finely chopped

1 tsp tomato purée/paste

1 tsp yellow mustard seeds

2 tsp garam masala

1 tsp ground turmeric

200g/7oz/1 cup dried red lentils

800ml/28fl oz/3½ cups vegetable stock

1 small cauliflower, broken into small florets

300g/11oz/6 cups spinach leaves

squeeze of lemon juice

a little chopped coriander/cilantro, for sprinkling

plain yogurt and naan breads, to serve (optional)

NOTE: Garam masala is a mellow blend of spices that is available in most supermarkets. It is a very useful mixture, with the advantage being that you don't have to buy separate jars of each spice.

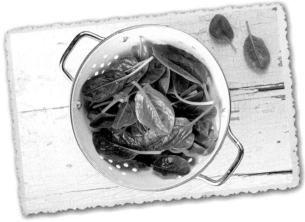

CHICKPEA AND BLACK-EYED BEAN CHILLI

I really like the texture of nutty chickpeas alongside the meatier black-eyed beans in this chilli, but you can use any combination of pulses or beans. Serve it with plain steamed rice and sour cream if you have some, or an avocado and tomato salsa.

SERVES 4

READY IN 40 MINUTES

rapeseed/canola oil, for cooking

1 large onion, sliced

1 garlic clove, finely chopped

1 heaped tsp tomato purée/paste

1 tsp ground coriander

1 tsp ground cumin

1 tsp chilli powder

400g/14oz/1¾ cups canned chopped tomatoes

115ml/4fl oz /½ cup vegetable stock

400g/14oz canned black-eyed beans, drained

400g/14oz canned chickpeas, drained

1 tbsp balsamic vinegar (or a couple of pinches of brown sugar)

small bunch of coriander/cilantro, roughly chopped

sea salt and freshly ground black pepper

lime wedges, to serve

sour cream, sprinkled with chilli powder, to serve (optional)

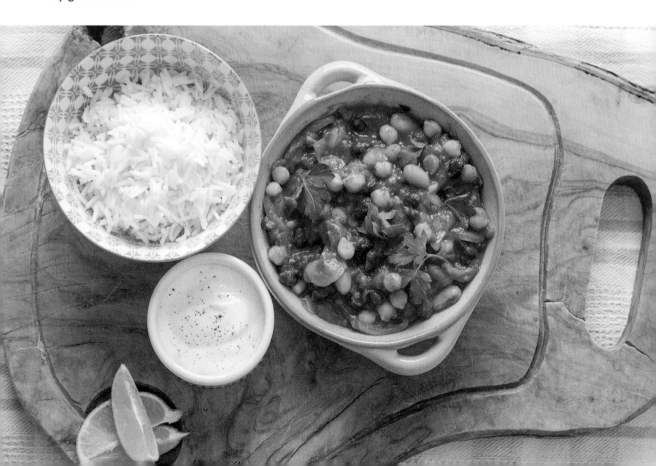

Heat a generous slug of oil in a casserole or deep frying pan over a medium heat. Add the onion and garlic and cook for 10 minutes until soft and beginning to colour.

Add the tomato purée/paste, ground coriander, cumin and chilli powder and stir over the heat for 1 minute, scraping the spices from the bottom of the pan as you go.

Pour in the tomatoes and stock and stir well. Add the black-eyed beans and chickpeas, bring to the boil, then reduce the heat and gently simmer for 15–20 minutes, stirring every so often.

Add the balsamic vinegar and most of the chopped coriander/cilantro and stir through gently. Season with salt and pepper and leave for a few minutes before serving to let the flavours develop. Scatter over the remaining coriander/cilantro. Serve with wedges of lime and a little sour cream with chilli powder sprinkled over, if you like.

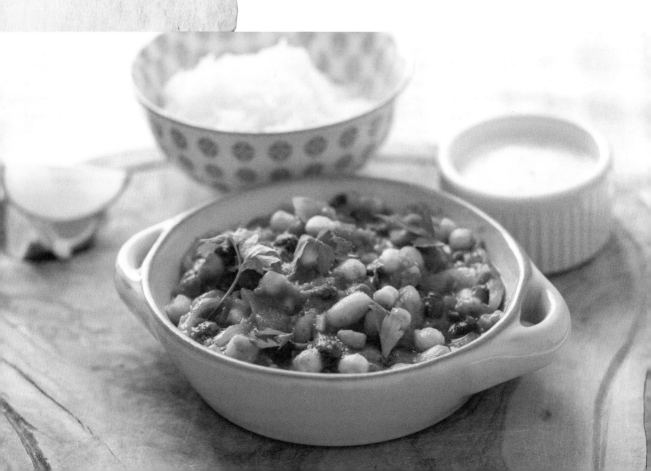

STUFFED COURGETTE FLOWERS

An early summer feast, these really are a celebration of courgettes/zucchini and their wonderful fresh flavour. The flowers can usually be found at a good greengrocer or local market when in season, but the best are those plucked from your garden and eaten on the same day. In this recipe, there is the option to add cream cheese to the mixture, which is delicious but not necessary if you're avoiding dairy; the stuffing is full of flavour as it is. I serve these with a drizzle of salsa verde (see page 94) and a big bowl of salad.

SERVES 4

READY IN **30** MINUTES

2 tbsp olive oil, plus extra if needed

3 courgettes/zucchini, cut into small cubes

4 garlic cloves, crushed

handful of basil leaves, chopped

handful of parsley leaves, chopped

zest of ½ lemon

3 tbsp cream cheese or soft goats' cheese (optional)

12 large courgette/zucchini flowers

225g/8oz/1¾ cups gluten-free plain/all-purpose flour

2 egg yolks

300ml/10½fl oz/1¼ cups cold sparkling water

sunflower oil, for cooking

sea salt and freshly ground black pepper

Heat the olive oil in a frying pan and cook the courgette/zucchini cubes for 5 minutes. Add the garlic and cook for a further 5 minutes, stirring and adding more oil if needed. Add the basil, parsley, lemon zest and some salt and pepper. Cook for another 2–3 minutes until the courgettes/zucchini are softened but still keep their shape. If using the cream cheese or goats' cheese, stir this in and take the mixture off the heat.

Carefully open up each flower and spoon in about 2 tablespoons of the stuffing mixture, being careful not to overfill. Gently press the flowers closed.

Place the flour in a large mixing bowl with a pinch of salt. Use a fork or whisk to beat in the egg yolks and sparkling water to form a batter.

Pour sunflower oil into a deep saucepan until about 12cm/4½in deep, and heat until hot enough to sizzle when you add a droplet of batter. Place the stuffed flowers into the batter, 2 or 3 at a time, turning to coat.

Carefully place the stuffed flowers in the hot oil and fry for 2 minutes until lightly golden, turning over in the oil once or twice. Drain on paper towels, sprinkle with salt and pepper and serve straight away.

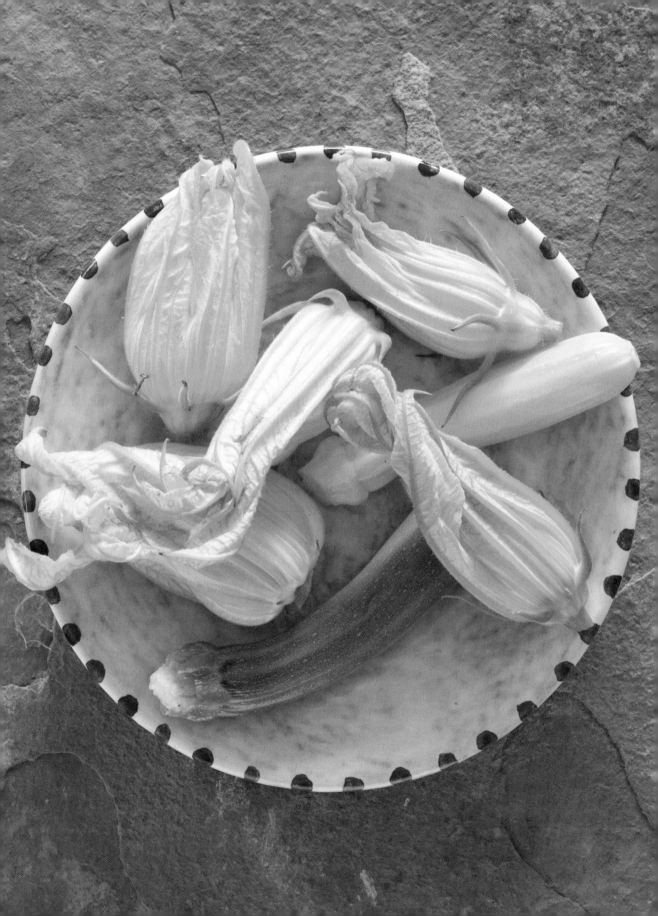

CELERIAC FRITTERS

READY IN **15** MINUTES

SERVES 4

1 celeriac (about 750g/1lb 10oz)

3 eggs, beaten

6 tbsp plain/all-purpose flour

1 tsp bicarbonate of soda/baking soda

juice of ½ lemon

3 tbsp crème fraîche

150ml/5fl oz/⅔ cup milk

few sprigs of dill, roughly chopped

rapeseed/canola oil and a knob of butter, for cooking

sea salt and freshly ground black pepper

sour cream, to serve

NOTE: The fritters are lovely with slices of grilled/broiled halloumi. Simply brush slices of halloumi with a little oil and place in a hot frying pan. Cook for 1 minute on each side until slightly golden.

Not the star of the kitchen catwalk, celeriac is often overlooked for its rough and knobbly appearance. Slice away the barky edges and shabby brown roots and the interior is pleasingly white and crisp. Raw, celeriac has a nutty, aniseed flavour that gives it away as celery's cousin and makes it a delicious addition to winter salads, coleslaws or a French remoulade. Here, it is grated into satisfying, light fritters, which can be served with sour cream or perhaps grilled/broiled halloumi.

Slice off and discard the celeriac's rough outer skin. Cut into manageable chunks and then grate, squeezing out as much liquid from the grated flesh as you can, before placing in a large bowl.

Pour the beaten eggs into a second bowl and add the flour, bicarbonate of soda/baking soda, lemon juice and crème fraîche and beat together well with a fork. Add a little salt and pepper, the milk and dill and beat again until smooth. Stir the grated celeriac into the batter mixture.

Heat about 4 tablespoons of rapeseed/canola oil in a frying pan with the butter and add a large tablespoon of the batter to the hot oil, flattening slightly with the back of the spoon (the oil and butter should sizzle when the fritter mixture is added).

Continue with more batter, to cook a few fritters at a time; fry for about 2 minutes until golden brown and slightly puffed. Flip the fritters over and cook until golden on the second side.

Remove the fritters to a plate and keep them warm while you cook the rest of the mixture in the same way, adding a little more oil to the pan as needed.

Serve while still warm with a little sour cream.

RED PEPPER, SPINACH AND FETA FRITTATA

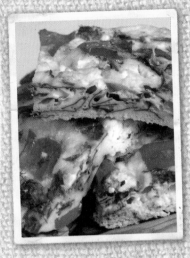

The sweetness of the peppers with salty feta and fragrant dill is a combination that really brings out each of the ingredients. Served warm in the evening with a gutsy salad or cold in your lunch box the next day, this is my favourite way to turn eggs into a feast.

Preheat the oven to 200°C/400°F/gas 6.

Place the peppers in a roasting tray with a little olive oil, salt and pepper. Toss together to coat the peppers in the oil and roast for 15 minutes until tender and soft but not burnt or blackened.

Meanwhile, shred the spinach leaves into ribbons. In a bowl, beat the eggs well with a fork and season with plenty of salt and pepper. Leave to one side.

Lightly grease a 30cm/12in round baking pan that is at least 2cm/1in deep, and line with baking parchment.

When the peppers are cooked, tip them into a bowl and mix through the spinach, dill and feta. Tip this mixture into the prepared pan, spreading it out across the bottom. Pour in the beaten eggs and stir very slightly to distribute the mixture evenly.

Place the pan toward the top of the oven and bake for 15 minutes until the eggs have set and the whole frittata is firm.

Leave to cool slightly and serve with green salad.

READY IN 40 MINUTES

SERVES 4

2 red peppers, deseeded and roughly chopped

olive oil, for cooking

50g/1¾oz/1 cup spinach leaves

8 large eggs

butter, for greasing

handful of dill, finely chopped

115g/4oz feta cheese, crumbled

sea salt and freshly ground black pepper

green salad, to serve

TUNISIAN PEPPERS AND EGGS

Cropping up on brunch menus in the last year or two, this Tunisian dish, known as Shakshuka, is equally worthy of a place in your kitchen on a weekday evening. The eggs are gently poached in a rich and smoky tomato sauce with plenty of herbs and spices. It's a perfect sharing dish – serve it in the pan it is cooked in so everyone can dive in.

READY IN 40 MINUTES

SERVES 4

rapeseed/canola oil, for cooking

1 red onion, sliced

2 red peppers, deseeded and sliced

1 yellow pepper, deseeded and sliced

2 garlic cloves, crushed

1 tsp ground cumin

1 tsp chilli powder

1 tsp paprika

1 tsp ground turmeric

1 tsp tomato purée/paste

800g/1lb 12oz/3½ cups canned chopped tomatoes

pinch of brown sugar, to taste (optional)

4 large eggs

sea salt and freshly ground black pepper

plain yogurt, to drizzle

handful of coriander/cilantro leaves, chopped

In a wide saucepan heat 2 tablespoons of oil over a medium heat. Add the onion and cook for about 5 minutes until just beginning to soften. Add the peppers and garlic and cook for a further 5 minutes, stirring frequently, until the vegetables are soft and slightly golden. If the pan looks dry, add another splash of oil.

Add the cumin, chilli powder, paprika, turmeric and tomato purée/paste to the pan and cook for 1 minute, stirring well. Pour in the tomatoes and bring to a gentle simmer. Add a little salt and pepper and leave the mixture to simmer gently for 10–15 minutes. Taste the sauce and if it's too sharp add a pinch or two of brown sugar.

Take the pan off the heat and make four small wells in the top of the tomato mixture. Gently crack an egg into each well and use a spoon to break up the whites of the egg slightly into the sauce, leaving the yolks whole. Return the pan to the heat, bring back to a gentle simmer and cover with a lid. Cook for 4–5 minutes until the yolks have just set. Spoon over a drizzle of yogurt and scatter over the coriander/cilantro before serving.

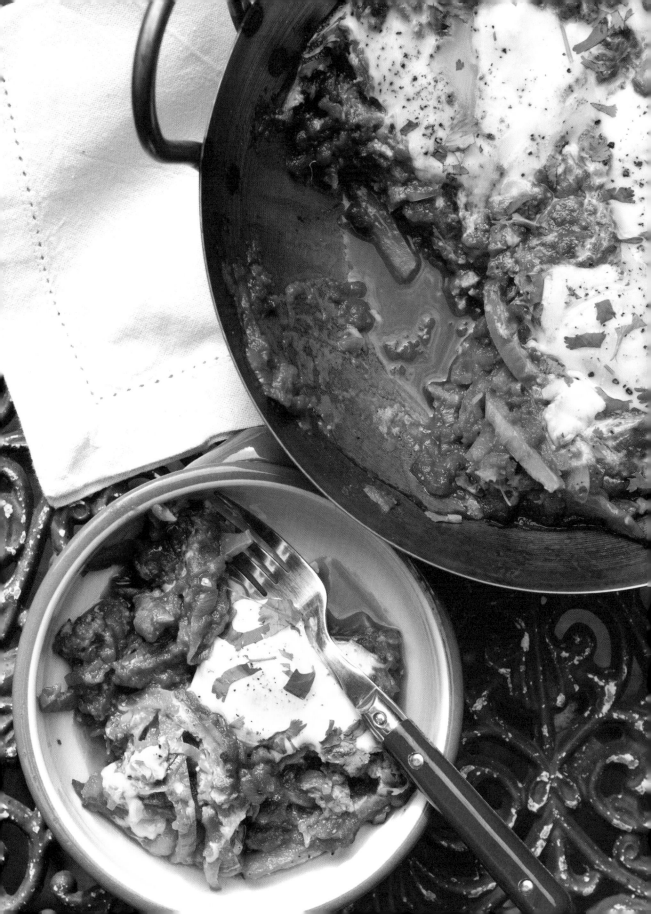

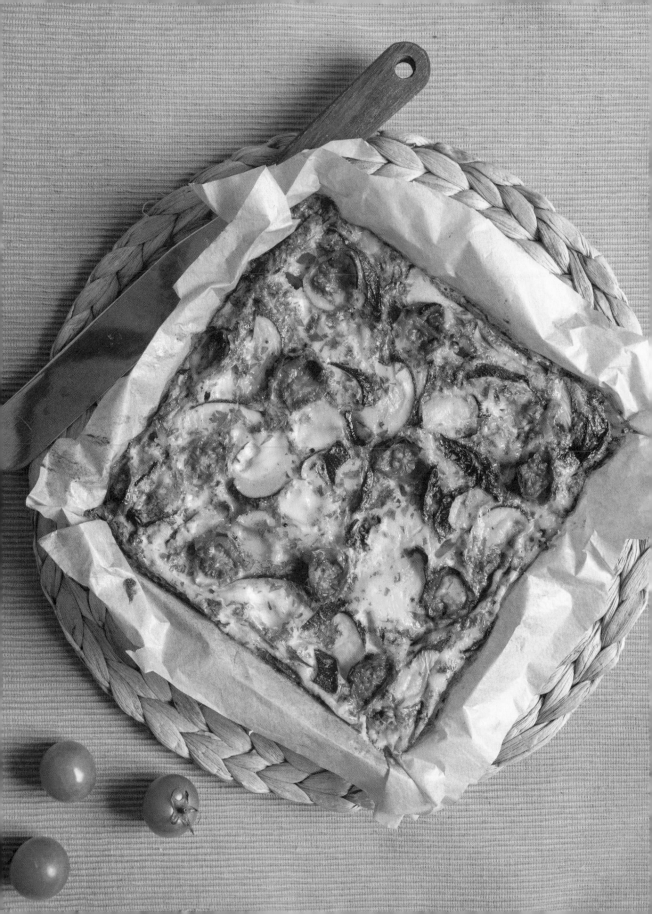

COURGETTE, CHERRY TOMATO AND GOATS' CHEESE FRITTATA

This is best during the summer months while courgettes/zucchini are in season, their sweet freshness making the frittata even more delicious. This is also a great lunch box recipe so if you find yourself with leftovers, make sure you wrap them up to take to work or school.

Preheat the oven to 190°C/375°F/gas 5.

Lightly grease a 20cm/8in square baking pan and line with baking parchment.

Cut the courgettes/zucchini in half lengthways and discard the ends. Cut into 5mm/¼in diagonal slices.

Place the courgettes/zucchini in a bowl with the garlic, oregano, olive oil and some salt and pepper and toss together. Spread out on a baking sheet and roast at the top of the oven for 15 minutes until cooked but still firm.

While the courgettes/zucchini are cooking beat the eggs together in a bowl using a fork, seasoning with salt and pepper. Once cooked, tip the courgettes/zucchini into the beaten eggs along with the parsley and mix well.

Pour this mixture into the prepared baking pan and then crumble the goats' cheese over the top, pushing the cheese lightly into the egg mixture. Do the same with the cherry tomatoes.

Turn the oven down to 180°C/350°F/gas 4 and bake on the middle shelf for 20 minutes until just set. Test by inserting a fork into the middle of the frittata; it should come out clean, with just a little egg clinging to the prongs.

READY IN 40 MINUTES

SERVES 4

500g/1lb 2oz small, young courgettes/zucchini

1 garlic clove, finely chopped

1 tsp dried oregano

2 tbsp olive oil

8 eggs

large handful of parsley, chopped

70g/2½oz soft goats' cheese

8 cherry tomatoes, halved

sea salt and freshly ground black pepper

NOTE: This is best served warm straight from the oven or at room temperature. If you plan to eat it another day, make sure you let it come to room temperature before serving.

MUSHROOM AND WILD RICE PILAF

This is a mild, aromatic pilaf with plenty of contrasting flavours and textures. You can use any combination of mushroom or rice varieties depending on your own preference and what you can find when you shop. I use a mix of dried and fresh mushrooms; the more variety the better, making the finished dish interesting, colourful and aromatic.

SERVES 4

READY IN 30 MINUTES

50g/1¾oz dried mushrooms (porcini, cep or shiitake, or a combination)

2 tbsp rapeseed/canola oil

6 black peppercorns

5 green cardamom pods

1 tsp cumin seeds

1 tsp yellow mustard seeds

1 onion, chopped

2 garlic cloves, crushed

200g/7oz fresh chestnut mushrooms, sliced

300ml/10½fl oz/1¼ cups vegetable stock

300g/10½oz/1½ cups wild rice (or a mixture of wild, brown and red Camargue rice)

50g/1¾oz/½ cup shelled pistachios, roughly chopped

juice of ½ lemon

handful of parsley, chopped, plus extra for sprinkling

sea salt and freshly ground black pepper

sour cream or yogurt, to serve (optional)

Begin by soaking the dried mushrooms. Tip them into a small bowl and pour over enough boiling water to cover.

While the mushrooms are soaking, heat the oil in a large casserole or frying pan. Add the peppercorns, cardamom pods, cumin and mustard seeds and fry for 2–3 minutes until the spices release lots of aroma and start to sizzle and pop. Add the onion and garlic to the pan and fry for 2 minutes.

Drain the soaked mushrooms, reserving the liquid, and slice. Add them to the pan along with the fresh mushrooms, stir well and cook over a low heat for 8–10 minutes. If the mixture seems dry, add a little of the soaking water. Meanwhile, heat the stock until gently simmering.

Stir in the rice and half of the pistachios and then pour over the soaking water and hot stock. Season with salt and pepper, cover with a lid and cook over a low heat for 12–15 minutes.

Remove the lid, taste to check the rice is tender and then add the lemon juice, parsley and more seasoning if needed. Serve topped with the remaining chopped pistachios, a little extra parsley and perhaps a drizzle of sour cream or yogurt, if you like.

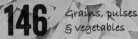

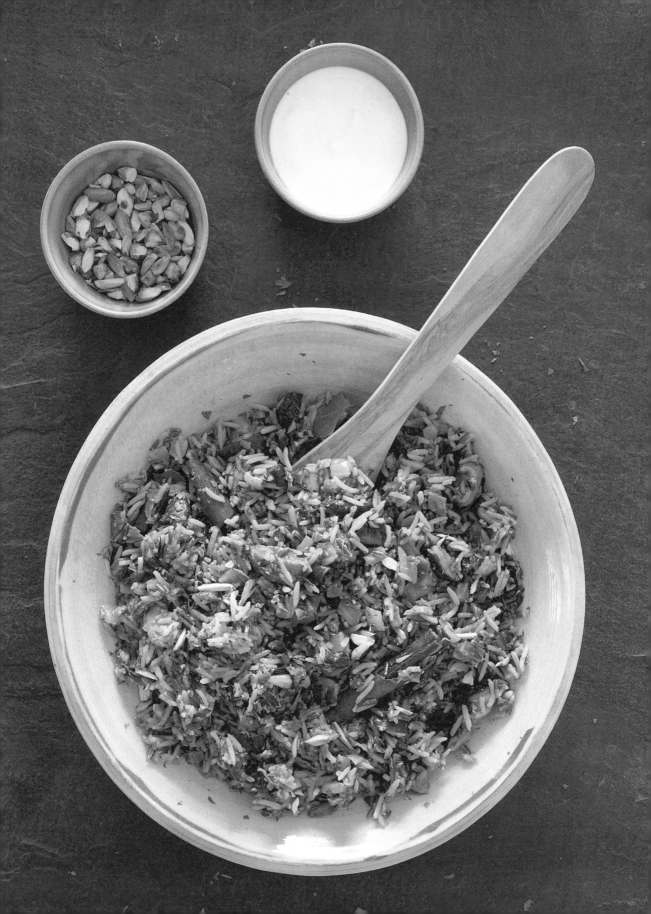

ROAST VEGETABLE PASTA WITH HERBS, CAPERS & PARMESAN

SERVES 4

1 yellow pepper, deseeded and sliced into strips

1 red pepper, deseeded and sliced into strips

1 large red onion, sliced

2 tsp dried rosemary

brown sugar, to taste

2 courgettes/zucchini, sliced diagonally

2 garlic cloves

350g/12oz dried pasta (conchiglie is lovely)

olive oil, for cooking

1 tbsp capers, roughly chopped

1 tbsp sun-dried tomatoes, sliced

handful of basil, roughly chopped

handful of parsley, roughly chopped

handful of chives, roughly chopped

85g/3oz Parmesan cheese

sea salt and freshly ground black pepper

pine nuts, toasted, to serve (optional)

Packed with colourful Mediterranean vegetables and herbs, this is a fresh, bright meal to end the day with. It sings of summer and long light evenings, hopefully spent eating outside. Enough to feed four, this is a perfect recipe to make for two, giving you a packed lunch for the following day.

Preheat the oven to 190°C/375°F/gas 5.

Toss the peppers and onion with 1 teaspoon of rosemary, a sprinkling of salt and pepper and a pinch of sugar. Spread out in a roasting tray.

Slice the courgettes/zucchini into chunky diagonal slices. Season as you did the peppers using the remaining rosemary, and place in a separate tray. Add the garlic cloves, still in their skins. Place both trays in the oven, with the peppers on the higher shelf, and cook for 25 minutes; check them every so often and toss to ensure even cooking.

Meanwhile, bring a large pan of salted water to the boil and cook the pasta for 10–12 minutes until al dente. Drain, return to the pan and toss some olive oil through it.

Take the roast vegetables out of the oven and squeeze the soft, cooked garlic flesh out of its skin. Discard the skin.

Add the garlic, capers, sun-dried tomatoes, basil, parsley and chives to the pasta and grate over half of the Parmesan. Toss really well before adding the roast vegetables and tossing once again.

Serve in large bowls with the remaining Parmesan grated or shaved on top and scattered with a few toasted pine nuts, if you like.

THAI VEGETABLE SLAW

This recipe involves very little cooking, and if you've got a good food processor, then you barely need to chop either. It's a fresh and crunchy pile of nutritious, colourful, shredded vegetables dressed with Thai flavours and topped with crunchy peanuts and shallots, if you have them in.

Preheat the oven to 190°C/375°F/gas 5.

Spread the peanuts out on a baking sheet and roast in the oven for 8–10 minutes until golden. Roughly chop and leave to one side.

Meanwhile, cut the cabbage, fennel, onion and pepper into manageable pieces, then shred them very finely; the easiest way to do this is in a food processor with a blade attachment but if you don't have one you can use a mandoline, grater or simply slice as finely as you can with a sharp knife.

Grate the carrot and courgette/zucchini into a large bowl and add the shredded vegetables, the coriander/cilantro leaves and most of the chopped peanuts.

To make the dressing, simply place all of the dressing ingredients, except the peanut butter, into a blender and blend until smooth and no pieces of garlic, ginger or chilli are visible. Add the peanut butter and blend for a few seconds to combine.

Tip the dressing out over the vegetables and mix thoroughly. Pile the salad onto plates and scatter any remaining peanuts on top of each plateful. If you like, scatter over a few crispy shallots, too.

READY IN 15 MINUTES

SERVES 4

55g/2oz/½ cup peanuts

¼ red cabbage

1 fennel bulb

1 red onion

1 red pepper

1 large carrot, peeled

1 courgette/zucchini

2 handfuls of coriander/cilantro leaves

small handful of crispy shallots, to serve (optional)

FOR THE DRESSING

2 garlic cloves

5cm/2in piece of root ginger, peeled and chopped

½ red chilli

juice of 2 limes

4 tbsp sesame oil

2 tbsp soy sauce

1 tbsp peanut butter

TIP: You can use any combination of raw vegetables in this recipe, such as beetroot/beets, butternut squash or even cauliflower and broccoli.

You can buy crispy shallots in most supermarkets and they add a delicious crunch to Thai-inspired salads.

BUTTERNUT SQUASH, CHESTNUT AND SAGE RISOTTO

A spoonful of autumn, this is a classic combination of comforting, earthy flavours to warm you as the evenings draw in. Roast the leftover butternut squash and throw it into a salad for lunch the next day.

READY IN 40 MINUTES

SERVES 4

- ½ butternut squash, peeled, deseeded and chopped into 1cm/½in dice
- olive oil, for cooking
- 115g/4oz/¾ cup vacuum-packed cooked chestnuts
- 85g/3oz/½ cup smoked bacon lardons
- knob of butter
- 1 celery stalk, finely chopped
- 1 onion, finely chopped
- 1 garlic clove, finely chopped
- 1l/35fl oz/4 cups vegetable stock
- 300g/10½oz/1½ cups Arborio rice
- 12 sage leaves, shredded
- 170ml/5½fl oz/ ⅔ cup white wine
- 4 slices pancetta, to serve (optional)
- 55g/2oz Parmesan cheese, grated
- squeeze of lemon juice
- handful of parsley, chopped
- sea salt and freshly ground black pepper

Preheat the oven to 200°C/400°F/gas 6.

Toss the butternut squash in a little olive oil, salt and pepper and spread on a baking sheet. Cook at the top of the oven for 10 minutes, then shake and turn the pieces of squash. Cook for a further 10 minutes until the squash is cooked through.

Meanwhile, crumble the chestnuts onto a second baking sheet, breaking them into small pieces. Place in the oven for 10 minutes until the pieces are toasted and slightly golden.

While the squash and chestnuts are cooking, put the bacon lardons in a large saucepan with a little olive oil and the butter. Cook over a medium heat for 3–4 minutes, then add the celery, onion and garlic. Cook for 5 minutes until softened but not coloured. Heat the stock in a pan, and leave to one side.

Tip the Arborio rice and sage into the pan with the lardon mixture. Stir well for 1 minute to coat the rice with oil and butter and then pour in the white wine. Let it simmer gently until the wine has been absorbed, then begin to add the stock, a couple of ladlefuls at a time, allowing the liquid to be absorbed by the rice in between each addition; keep stirring throughout.

When nearly all of the stock has been absorbed, taste to check if the rice is cooked. It should be al dente (cooked, but with a little bite). If not, add more stock and cook for a little longer. If you would like to add pancetta, fry the slices in a little olive oil for 3–4 minutes until crispy, and leave to one side.

Add the butternut squash and chestnut pieces along with the Parmesan, lemon juice and a little salt and pepper. Add a little more stock if needed; the texture should be relaxed and slightly oozing. Leave to rest for a few minutes before scattering over the parsley. Top with the pancetta, if using.

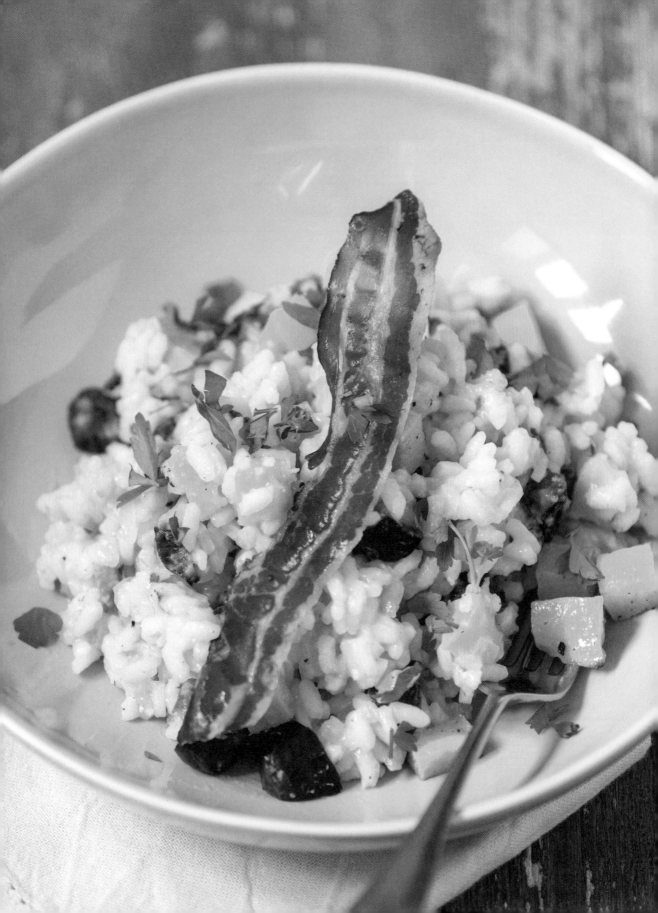

SWEETCORN PANCAKES WITH AVOCADO SALSA

Bright and colourful, this fresh recipe makes a delicious light supper. It's a good weekend brunch dish, too, which you could serve topped with a poached egg for each person.

SERVES 4

READY IN 20 MINUTES

3 eggs

115g/4oz/¾ cup plain/all-purpose flour

1 tsp baking powder

115ml/4fl oz/½ cup crème fraîche

170g/6oz/1 cup canned sweetcorn

bunch of coriander/cilantro, chopped

small bunch of spring onions/scallions, sliced

rapeseed/canola oil, for frying

sea salt and freshly ground black pepper

lime wedges, to serve

FOR THE SALSA

4 tomatoes, diced

1 red onion, diced

1 ripe avocado, peeled, pitted and diced

1 red chilli, deseeded and finely chopped

1 garlic clove, crushed

juice of 1 lime

2 tbsp olive oil

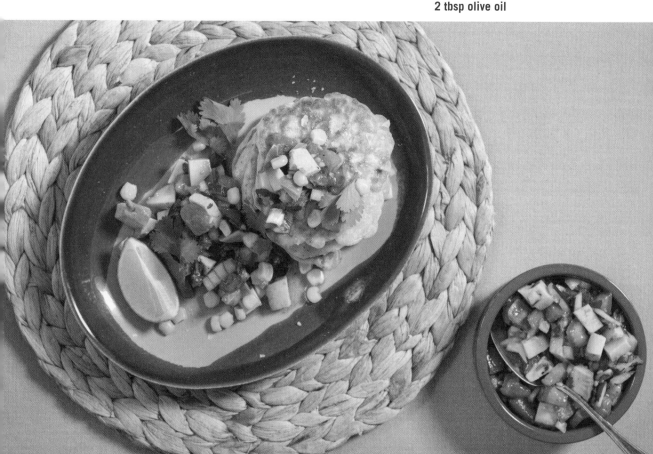

Start off by making the pancake batter. Place the eggs, flour, baking powder, crème fraîche and two-thirds of the sweetcorn in a blender. Blend for about 30 seconds until smooth. Tip the batter into a bowl and then stir in the remaining sweetcorn, half of the coriander/cilantro, the spring onions/scallions and a pinch of salt. Leave to one side while you make the salsa.

To make the salsa, combine the tomatoes, onion, avocado, chilli and garlic in a bowl. Add the lime juice, olive oil and some salt and pepper. Stir well and then add most of the remaining chopped coriander/cilantro. (If you have any extra sweetcorn left you can add this to the salsa, too.)

To cook the pancakes, heat a little rapeseed/canola oil in a frying pan and when sizzling, drop in 2–3 large tablespoons of batter at a time, letting each spread out to form small round pancakes. Cook for about 2 minutes, then flip over to cook for a further 2 minutes, until nicely golden brown. Keep the pancakes warm while you cook the rest of the batter.

Once all of the pancakes are cooked, top with the salsa and the remaining coriander/cilantro. Serve with wedges of lime to squeeze over.

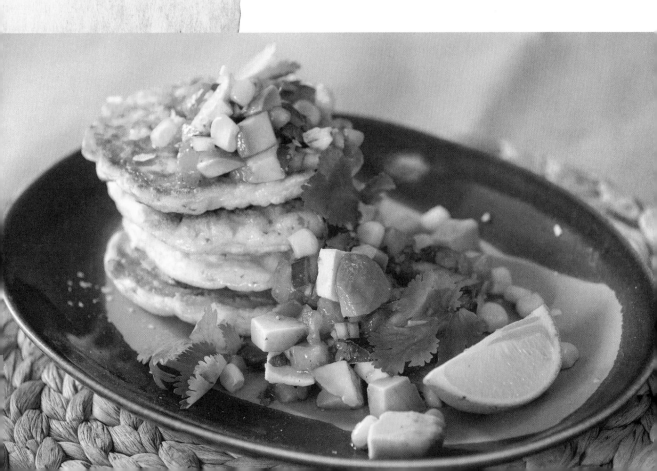

GREEK STUFFED RED PEPPERS WITH COUSCOUS AND FETA

SERVES 4

2 large red peppers

olive oil, for cooking

170g/6oz/1 cup couscous

4 tomatoes, diced

1 red onion, finely chopped

2 garlic cloves, finely chopped

24 pitted black olives, halved

handful of mint, roughly chopped

handful of dill, roughly chopped

handful of parsley, roughly chopped

juice of 1 lemon

115g/4oz feta cheese

sea salt and freshly ground black pepper

green salad, to serve

NOTE: You could use quinoa instead of couscous in this recipe. Place 170g/6oz/1 cup quinoa in a large saucepan. Cover with water, bring to the boil and simmer gently for 10–15 minutes until the grains are cooked but still have a little bite. Drain in a colander and continue as for the couscous stuffing above.

These stuffed peppers are wonderfully simple to make and delicious warm or cold with plenty of fresh green salad. If you're avoiding gluten then cooked quinoa works as a delicious alternative to the couscous, the almost nutty grains offering lots of texture.

Preheat the oven to 200°C/400°F/gas 6.

Using a sharp knife, halve the peppers, being careful to slice through the green stalk too, in order to leave both halves with a piece of stalk attached. Remove and discard the seeds and any white pith.

Place on a baking sheet, drizzle with a little olive oil and bake at the top of the oven for 20 minutes.

Meanwhile, prepare the stuffing. Tip the couscous into a bowl, add a little salt and pepper and 1 tablespoon of olive oil. Pour 150ml/5fl oz/⅔ cup boiling water over the couscous, stir well and cover with a plate. Leave to one side for 10 minutes and then use a fork to fluff up the couscous, separating all of the grains.

Add the tomatoes, red onion, garlic, olives, mint, dill, parsley and lemon juice and mix well. Taste and add a little more salt, pepper, olive oil or lemon juice as needed. Lastly, crumble the feta into the bowl and gently stir through the mixture.

Remove the peppers from the oven and divide the couscous filling between them, pressing down lightly. Drizzle over a little more olive oil and return to the top of the oven for 5 minutes to warm through. Serve with green salad.

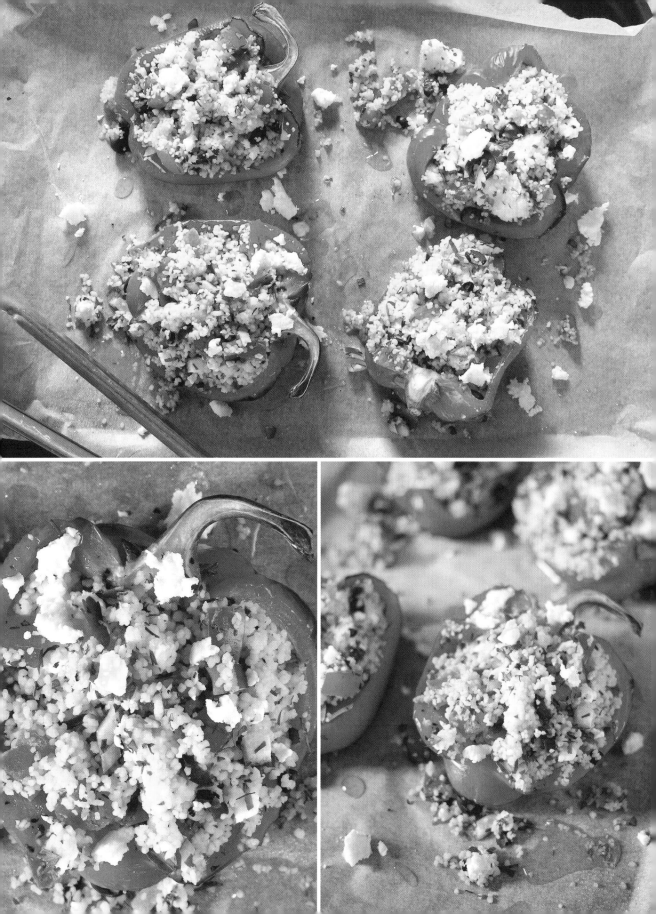

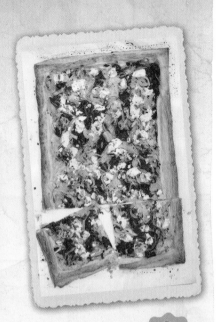

LEEK, SPINACH AND FETA TART

An impressive creation for the middle of the kitchen table, this tart is very quick to make when you get home from work. Buy fresh sheets of puff pastry rather than frozen blocks to speed up the cooking time, and try replacing the feta with a soft blue cheese if you prefer.

SERVES 4

READY IN **40** MINUTES

30g/1oz/2 tbsp butter

2 leeks, finely sliced

rapeseed/canola oil, for cooking

1 garlic clove, crushed

1 tbsp thyme leaves

300g/10½oz/6 cups spinach leaves

1 sheet ready-rolled puff pastry

115g/4oz feta cheese

a little milk, for brushing

sea salt and freshly ground black pepper

green salad, to serve

Preheat the oven to 220°C/425°F/gas 7.

Melt the butter in a saucepan with a little oil and add the leeks, garlic and thyme. Cover with a lid and fry over a low heat for 10 minutes until softened but not coloured. Season with salt and pepper.

Meanwhile, wash the spinach leaves and place in another pan over a medium heat. Cover with a lid and cook for 2 minutes until the leaves have wilted. Tip into a colander and drain well, squeezing out as much moisture as you can.

Lightly grease a baking sheet with oil and line with baking parchment. Unroll the puff pastry and place on the baking parchment. Using a sharp knife, lightly score a 1cm/½in border all the way round the edge of the pastry, being careful not to cut all the way through.

Spread the cooked leek mixture and spinach over the pastry, keeping within the border. Crumble the feta cheese over the top of the vegetables, filling in any gaps. Season with a little more pepper and brush the edges of pastry with a little milk.

Bake for 20 minutes on the top shelf of the oven until the pastry edges are risen and golden and the feta has started to brown.

Serve hot or cold with a bowl of green salad.

ASPARAGUS AND TARRAGON RISOTTO

This classic dish makes the most of fresh asparagus, which is at its finest in spring and early summer. Apart from the freshest asparagus you can find, all you need is a strong arm for stirring and a little patience. It's delicious served with a peppery rocket/ arugula salad.

Cut off and discard the woody ends of the asparagus and slice the remaining stems into thin discs.

Heat the oil in a heavy based saucepan over a low heat. Add the shallots and celery and fry gently for about 5 minutes until softened. Keep the heat low to stop the vegetables colouring.

Add the rice, asparagus and half of the tarragon. Stir well over a medium heat for a minute or so to coat the grains of rice in oil.

Pour in the white wine, bring to a simmer and stir until the liquid has been absorbed. Meanwhile, warm the vegetable stock. Add a ladleful or two at a time to the risotto, stirring well between additions and waiting for the stock to be absorbed before adding the next ladleful.

After most of the stock has been absorbed, taste the rice to test whether it's cooked. The grains should be al dente (cooked, but with a little bite). Take the pan off the heat, season well with salt and pepper and add the remaining tarragon and lemon juice.

Leave to rest for a minute or two and serve with the goats' cheese crumbled over the top.

READY IN
30
MINUTES

SERVES 4

large bunch of asparagus

2 tbsp rapeseed/canola oil

2 banana shallots, finely chopped

1 celery stalk, finely chopped

300g/10½oz/1½ cups risotto rice

handful of tarragon leaves, roughly chopped

225ml/8fl oz/1 cup white wine

700ml/24fl oz/3 cups vegetable stock

squeeze of lemon juice

85g/3oz soft goats' cheese

sea salt and freshly ground black pepper

NOTE: You could replace the goats' cheese with shavings of Parmesan or try adding other fresh herbs in place of tarragon, such as parsley or chives. You could use chicken stock instead of vegetable stock if you prefer.

BROAD BEAN, PEA AND FREEKEH RISOTTO

A nutty grain, cultivated in the Middle East, freekeh lends itself well to Middle Eastern pilafs and salads such as tabbouleh. Cooked slowly for a risotto it absorbs lots of flavour and creates an earthy and textured dish.

SERVES 4

READY IN 30 MINUTES

rapeseed/canola oil, for cooking

1 large onion, finely chopped

1 garlic clove, finely chopped

1l/35fl oz/4 cups vegetable stock

250g/9oz/1½ cups freekeh

handful of parsley, chopped

handful of dill, chopped

250g/9oz/1½ cups shelled fresh broad/fava beans

170g/6oz/2 cups fresh shelled peas

juice of ½ lemon

100g/3½oz soft goats' cheese

sea salt and freshly ground black pepper

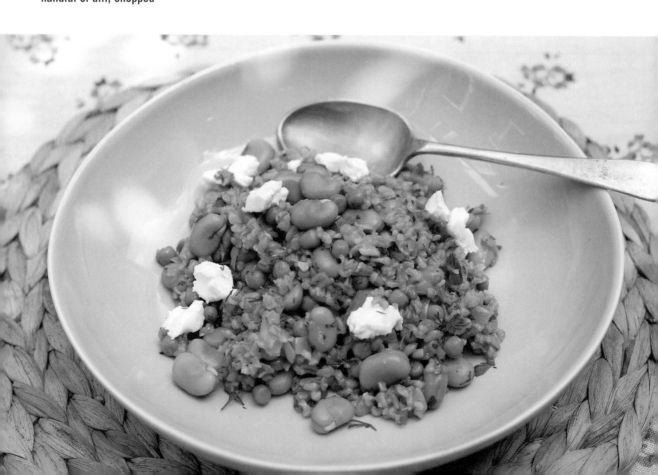

Heat a generous slug of oil in a large saucepan and add the onion and garlic. Cook gently for about 5 minutes until the onion has softened and is translucent. Meanwhile, heat the stock until bubbling.

Rinse the freekeh under cold running water, drain and add to the pan with the onion and garlic. Stir well to coat in the oil and then add a couple of ladles of hot stock. Stir over a low heat until the stock has almost all been absorbed. Add 2 more ladlefuls of stock and repeat, allowing the liquid to be absorbed in between additions. Keep doing this, a few ladles at a time, until the freekeh is cooked but still al dente (cooked, but with a little bite); it will take about 15 minutes.

Stir in the chopped herbs and some salt and pepper.

While the freekeh is cooking, cook the broad/fava beans and peas in a pan of boiling, salted water for about 2 minutes. Drain and cool under cool running water and then shell the beans by popping each one out of its pale green outer skin. Stir the beans into the freekeh along with the peas and lemon juice.

Return to the heat for 1–2 minutes, adding a little more stock if the mixture looks dry. Taste to check the seasoning and serve with the goats' cheese crumbled over the top.

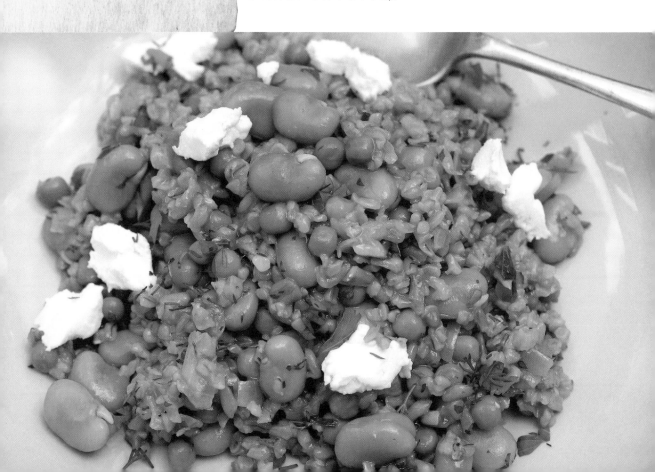

QUINOA, COURGETTE AND HERB CAKES

These little cakes are free of gluten and dairy if you're sensitive to either. The quinoa gives them a firm, nutty texture, which is delicious with the fresh herbs and courgette/zucchini. Dipped in a little garlic mayonnaise, chilli jam or tomato chutney, they're wonderful.

SERVES 4

READY IN 30 MINUTES

140g/5oz/1 cup quinoa

300g/10½oz courgette/zucchini, grated

3 spring onions/scallions, sliced

1 garlic clove, crushed

handful of mint leaves, shredded

handful of parsley leaves, chopped

10 sun-dried tomatoes, chopped

juice of ½ lemon

55g/2oz/½ cup cornflour/cornstarch

1 egg

rapeseed/canola oil, for frying

sea salt and freshly ground black pepper

garlic mayonnaise, chilli jam or tomato chutney, to serve

green salad, to serve

Tip the quinoa into a small saucepan and cover with 300ml/10½fl oz/ 1¼ cups of cold water. Bring to the boil, cover with a lid and cook for about 5 minutes until all the water has been absorbed and the quinoa is cooked. Turn out into a bowl and leave to one side to cool.

Meanwhile, place the grated courgette/zucchini in the bowl of a food processor with the spring onions/scallions, garlic, mint, parsley, sun-dried tomatoes, lemon juice and cornflour/cornstarch. Crack the egg straight into the mixture, add the quinoa, and season with salt and pepper. Blend for about 30 seconds to mix the ingredients thoroughly and to form a thick paste. Tip the mixture out into a bowl and taste to check the seasoning.

Heat about 5mm/¼in rapeseed/canola oil in a large frying pan until the oil is hot enough to sizzle loudly when you drop in a tiny bit of the courgette/ zucchini mixture.

Drop a heaped tablespoon of the mixture into the hot oil, flattening slightly with the back of the spoon to form round patties. Repeat until you have 3–4 cakes in the pan at the same time, or as many as your pan will fit comfortably, with room to turn.

After 3–4 minutes the underside of the cakes should be nicely golden and holding their shape. Gently flip them over and cook until the second side is golden. Lift the cakes out of the oil onto some paper towels and keep warm. Repeat until all of the mixture has been used; you should end up with 12–14 cakes. Serve the cakes warm with green salad and your choice of dip.

NOTE: To make a very quick garlic mayonnaise or aioli, add 2 crushed garlic cloves to 4 tbsp good-quality mayonnaise along with a squeeze of lemon juice. Season with freshly ground black pepper and, if needed, a little sea salt.

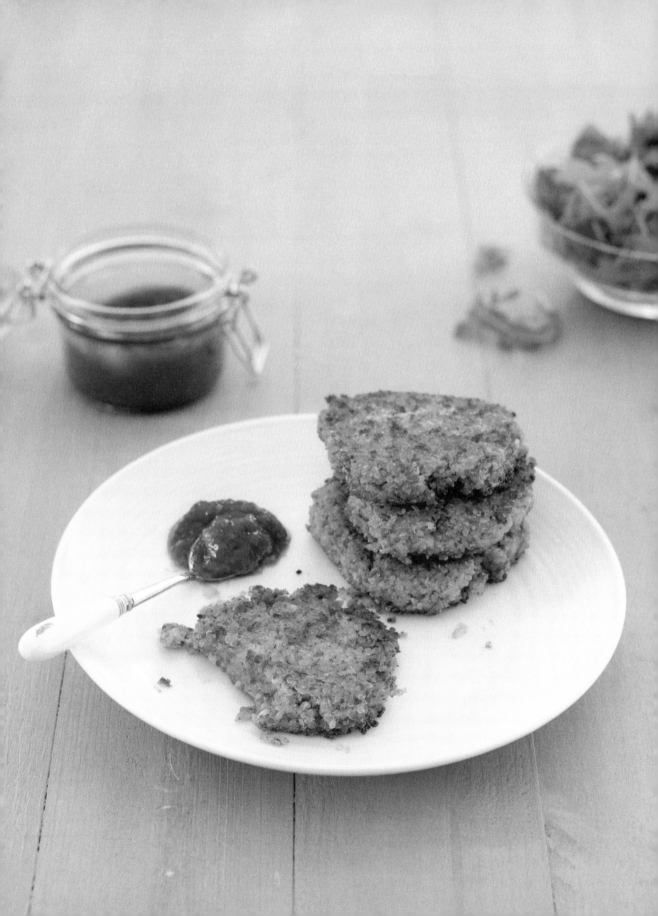

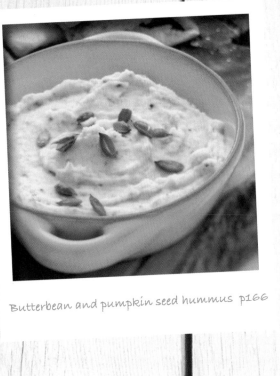

Butterbean and pumpkin seed hummus p166

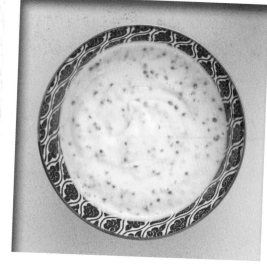

Grainy mustard mayonnaise p169

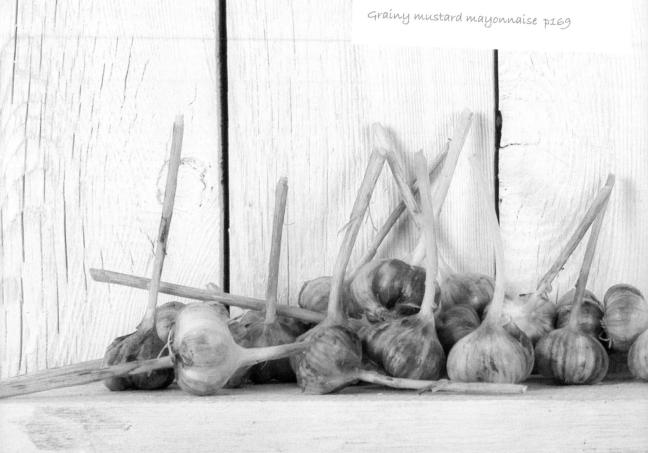

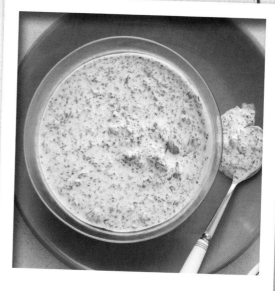

Watercress sauce p168

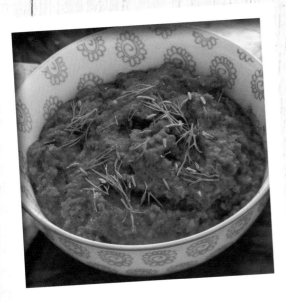

Beetroot and walnut dip p167

DIPS, SAUCES & DRESSINGS

SMOKY SQUASH, RED PEPPER AND GARLIC DIP

A jar of roasted peppers is a useful cupboard staple, and saves you having to roast and peel peppers if you are rushed for time.

SERVES 4

READY IN 40 MINUTES

1 small butternut squash, peeled, deseeded and chopped

100ml/3½fl oz/scant ½ cup olive oil (or half olive and rapeseed/canola oil), plus extra for drizzling

2 large red peppers (either fresh or ready-roasted from a jar)

4 garlic cloves, unpeeled

1 tsp smoked paprika, plus extra for sprinkling

½ tsp chilli powder

splash of red or white wine vinegar

sea salt and freshly ground black pepper

Preheat the oven to 190°C/375°F/gas 5.

Put the butternut squash in a large bowl with a little of the oil, salt and pepper and toss until coated. If you are using fresh peppers, deseed and cut into chunks. Add them to the butternut squash and coat in the oil, too. Spread out the vegetables on a baking sheet and add the garlic cloves, still in their skins. Roast for 25–30 minutes until the squash is soft and easily squashed with the back of a fork.

As soon as the peppers come out of the oven, pop them in a plastic bag and seal. Leave them to cool a little before peeling.

Meanwhile, squeeze the roast garlic out of its skin and place the flesh in a food processor with the butternut squash, peeled peppers (or jarred peppers), smoked paprika and chilli powder. Blend until combined but not completely smooth (it's nice to keep a bit of texture). Slowly pour in the olive oil and blend until combined. Add the vinegar and some salt and pepper and give it a final blend before tipping out into a bowl. Sprinkle over a little extra smoked paprika to serve.

NOTE: Homemade dips have become a bit of an obsession of mine and a rather substantial part of my diet. Despite the staggering array of pre-made options that are available to buy, none are as good as those you can make at home, given a little spare time and a decent blender. These recipes are not only bright and vibrant but pack a flavourful punch, which will definitely persuade you to keep making your own.

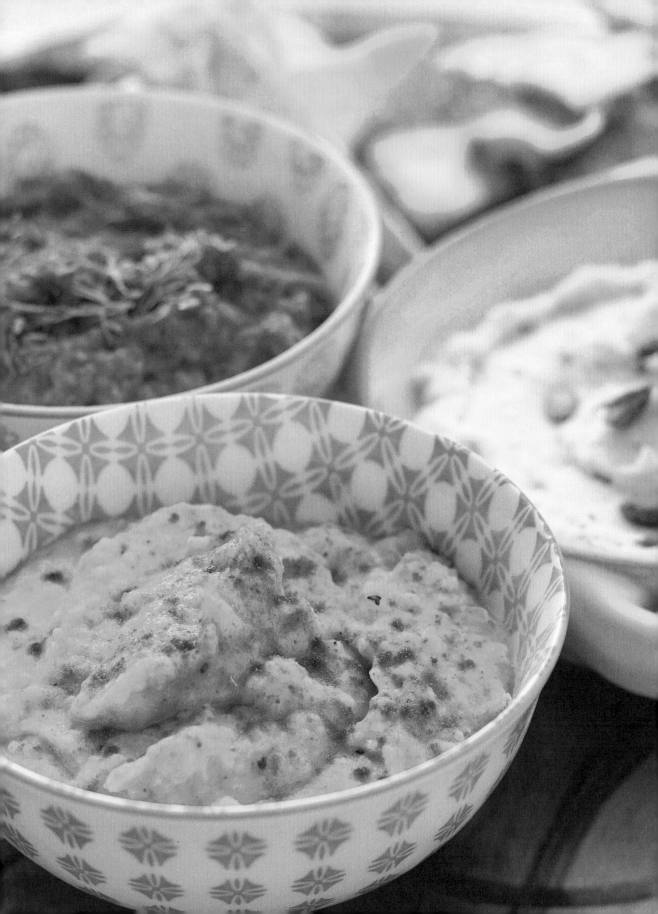

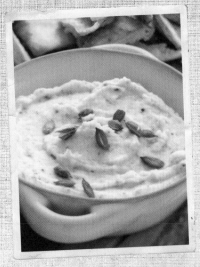

BUTTER BEAN AND PUMPKIN SEED HUMMUS

Creamy, soft butter/lima beans make a quick and protein-packed dip. Vary the seeds according to what you have in; sunflower seeds would work well in place of pumpkin seeds, for example.

SERVES 4

READY IN
15
MINUTES

30g/1oz pumpkin seeds

400g/14oz canned butter/lima beans, drained, liquid reserved

½ tsp ground cumin

½ tsp paprika

1 tbsp tahini

juice of ½ a lemon

100ml/3½fl oz/scant ½ cup olive oil

sea salt and freshly ground black pepper

Preheat the oven to 200°C/400°F/gas 6.

Spread the pumpkin seeds on a baking sheet and roast for 8–10 minutes until golden.

Meanwhile, place the butter/lima beans in a food processor with the ground cumin, paprika, tahini, lemon juice and olive oil and blend to the texture of a coarse hummus. If the dip is too thick, add a little of the reserved butter/lima bean liquid and blend again.

Taste and add salt and pepper as needed. Add the roasted pumpkin seeds, keeping a few back to sprinkle on top. Blend again for a few seconds to break up and incorporate the seeds and serve with the remaining pumpkin seeds on top.

NOTE: To make your own pitta bread chips to scoop up your dips, open out a few pitta breads like butterflies and cut into triangles. Put the triangles on a large baking sheet and drizzle with plenty of olive or rapeseed/canola oil and add some salt and pepper. Toss together so that all of the triangles have a dousing of oil and seasoning. Bake at 180°C/350°F/gas 4 for 15 minutes, shaking the sheet every few minutes so that they bake evenly.

BEETROOT AND WALNUT DIP

Choose the cooked beetroot/beets that comes in packs for this, rather than the pickled options that taste mostly of vinegar. It's a pretty flexible recipe; you can play around with different nuts and seeds depending on what you have in the cupboard; pistachios work well in place of the walnuts, for example.

Preheat the oven to 190°C/375°F/gas 5.

Spread the walnuts out on a baking sheet and roast for 8–10 minutes until the nuts are lightly golden. Tip the walnuts into a food processor and blitz until finely chopped and then tip out into a bowl.

Meanwhile, place the beetroot/beets into the food processor with the cumin, most of the dill, lemon juice and yogurt. Blend for 1 minute until smooth, then pour in the olive oil with the processor still running.

Tip in the ground walnuts, add some salt and pepper, then blend again to combine. Sprinkle over the remaining dill to serve.

SERVES 4

READY IN 15 MINUTES

100g/3½oz/¾ cup walnuts

400g/14oz cooked beetroot/beets, drained and roughly chopped

½ tsp ground cumin

handful of dill, chopped

juice of 1 lemon

100ml/3½fl oz/½ cup plain yogurt

50ml/2fl oz/¼ cup olive oil

sea salt and freshly ground black pepper

NOTE: Roast your own beetroot/beets if you have the time as it adds real depth of flavour.

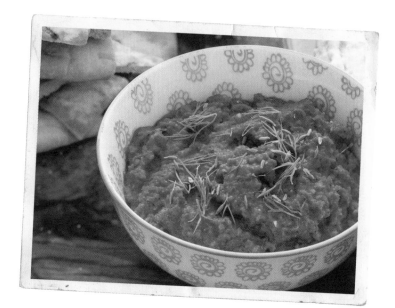

WATERCRESS SAUCE

SERVES 4

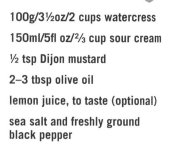

100g/3½oz/2 cups watercress

150ml/5fl oz/⅔ cup sour cream

½ tsp Dijon mustard

2–3 tbsp olive oil

lemon juice, to taste (optional)

sea salt and freshly ground black pepper

This is a great sauce to use throughout the warm summer months – serve it as an accompaniment to cold poached salmon, to dress a potato salad or in a bowl at a barbecue to spoon over chargrilled meats.

Discard any thick stalks from the watercress and place the leaves into a blender. Add all of the remaining ingredients and blend for 2–3 minutes until smooth. Taste to check the seasoning, adding a touch of lemon juice or more salt or pepper if needed.

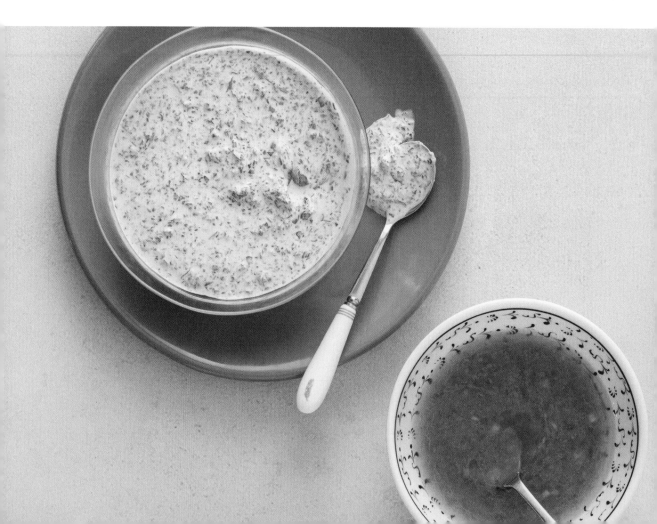

GRAINY MUSTARD MAYONNAISE

This is such a delicious addition to a whole raft of dishes; use in a steak sandwich, as a dip for some sweet potato fries or use it to make a herby potato salad. The addition of mustard to the egg yolks at the beginning stabilizes the sauce, making it less likely to curdle. You can use an electric beater if you like, but I find it just as easy to make with a hand-held whisk.

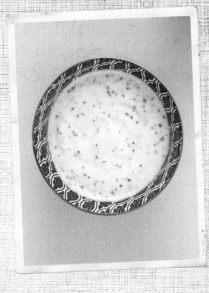

2 egg yolks

1 garlic clove, crushed

2 tsp wholegrain mustard

200ml/7fl oz /¾ cup rapeseed/ canola oil

1 tsp white wine vinegar

sea salt and freshly ground black pepper

Place the egg yolks in a bowl with the garlic, mustard and a pinch of salt and pepper. Lightly whisk together and slowly begin to pour in the oil, a few drops at a time, whisking all the time.

As the mayonnaise starts to emulsify (emulsify is to mix together without splitting) you can add the oil in a steady stream, still whisking, until all the oil has been incorporated. Stir in the vinegar and taste to check the seasoning, adding a little more salt and pepper if needed.

NOTE: Once made, you can add your own favourite additions to the mayonnaise. Tarragon, parsley and chives are very good, for instance, or try adding a pinch of paprika or chilli powder. You can also replace the wholegrain mustard with Dijon mustard, if you prefer. This mayonnaise should last for up to five days if kept in a jar in the fridge.

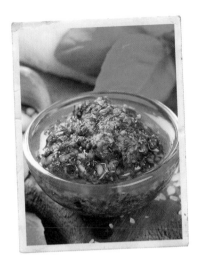

CLASSIC PESTO

This is so simple it should be stamped in every cook's memory! When freshly made, pesto is vibrant, nutty and bright; a completely different sauce to its pre-made jarred cousin. I always toast the pine nuts, which gives a wonderful depth to the finished flavour.

Pesto is, of course, a delicious sauce for pasta but it is also great as a dressing for warm roasted vegetables and potatoes, spread on toast or in a sandwich, used as a dip, or to top fish and chicken before grilling/broiling or baking.

SERVES 8

READY IN **15** MINUTES

55g/2oz/½ cup pine nuts

85g/3oz/1½ cups basil leaves

2 garlic cloves, peeled

55g/2oz Parmesan cheese, grated

200ml/7fl oz/¾ cup extra virgin olive oil

squeeze of lemon juice

freshly ground black pepper

Preheat the oven to 180°C/350°F/gas 4.

Spread the pine nuts out on a baking sheet and roast for 8–10 minutes until golden. Tip the roasted nuts into the bowl of a food processor or blender. Add the basil along with the garlic and Parmesan. Blend for a few seconds and, with the motor running, pour in the olive oil to form a thick green sauce. Add a little pepper and the lemon juice and taste the sauce. It's unlikely to need any salt as Parmesan is very salty, but you may need more pepper or lemon juice. This should last for up to five days if kept in the fridge.

NOTE: Using these quantities you can experiment with an array of herbs, seeds and nuts either to include your own favourite ingredients or simply to make use of what you might find in the cupboard or garden. These are a few of my favourite combinations: walnut and rocket/arugula, almond and parsley, pumpkin seed and basil, and pistachio and chive.

DIJON VINAIGRETTE

No one makes a better vinaigrette dressing than my Dad and I include his recipe here for you; he uses plenty of Dijon mustard, runny honey and lots of seasoning. I always make a big batch; it stores well if kept in a jar in the fridge. Making it in a jar saves on both whisking and washing up.

Measure all the ingredients into a screw-top jar. Shake as hard as you can to thoroughly combine and emulsify the dressing. This should last for up to five days if kept in the fridge.

SERVES 4

2 tsp Dijon mustard

2 tsp runny honey

3 tbsp white wine vinegar

3 tbsp rapeseed/canola oil

3 tbsp olive oil

sea salt and freshly ground black pepper

TIP: To this basic vinaigrette you can add other ingredients such as a crushed garlic clove, very finely chopped herbs or a grating of lemon zest.

GINGER AND SHALLOT DRESSING

I love to use this dressing with autumnal roasted vegetables or with bitter leaf salads of chicory/Belgian endive or radicchio, served alongside smoked fish or rich, gamey meats.

Put the grated ginger in a screw-top jar with the shallot. Add the remaining ingredients and shake to combine thoroughly. Taste to check the seasoning and add a little more sugar, lemon juice, salt or pepper if needed.

(Pictured on page 168)

SERVES 4

2cm/¾in piece of root ginger, peeled and grated

1 small shallot, finely chopped

1 tbsp soy sauce

2 tbsp sherry vinegar

squeeze of lemon juice

4 tbsp olive oil

pinch of sugar

sea salt and freshly ground black pepper

INDEX

ACKNOWLEDGEMENTS

This book wouldn't have happened without a huge amount of support and encouragement from friends, colleagues and family. You know who you are, but Ed you deserve the biggest thank you for patiently coping with the photo shoots and last minute panics. Hussy and Charlotte, your kitchen is where it all started; Diana, your positivity is tireless; and Margie, your beautiful crockery was a godsend. Andrew Crowley, Rebecca Woods, Becky Alexander, Cerys Hughes, Viki Ottewill and Geoff Borin – it is your brilliant professionalism that made this happen and I can't thank you enough.

AUTHOR BIOGRAPHY

Katriona MacGregor is a British cook and food writer who has written a weekly recipe column for the *Telegraph*. After years cooking for private clients and in restaurants she turned her hand to recipe writing, focusing on her love of British flavours and ingredients. Her personal experiences of stress, fatigue and autoimmune thyroid disease have led her to create recipes that are simple to make but focus on wholesome ingredients and nutritious eating. She lives in rural Oxfordshire, working at The Cookery School at Daylesford Organic.

PHOTOGRAPHY CREDITS

Hugh Carter: 62, 63, 89, 116

Andrew Crowley: 5 (top and middle), 9, 10–11, 13, 16 (left), 17 (left and right), 23, 24, 26, 27, 30, 35, 38, 41, 42, 48 (left and right), 49 (left and right), 51, 52, 53, 61, 65, 66, 69, 70, 72, 73, 74 (right), 75 (left), 77, 81, 84, 85, 91, 92, 93, 95, 101, 102 (right), 103 (right), 105, 106, 112, 115, 120, 127, 128, 130 (left and right), 131 (left and right), 133, 136, 137, 139, 144, 147, 151, 152, 153, 156, 161, 162 (left and right), 163 (left and right), 165, 166, 167, 168, 169

John Lawrence: 5 (bottom), 75 (right), 98, 102 (left), 109 (all), 155

Clara Molden: 59, 158, 159

Heathcliff O'Malley: 1, 2, 16 (right), 19, 33 (all), 45, 87, 103 (left), 110, 123 (all), 143

Martin Pope: 124, 141

David Rose: 55 (all), 74 (left), 78, 119, 134

All other photos: Shutterstock.com

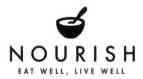

NOURISH
EAT WELL, LIVE WELL

Here at Nourish we're all about wellbeing through food and drink – irresistible dishes with a serious good-for-you factor. If you want to eat and drink delicious things that set you up for the day, suit any special diets, keep you healthy and make the most of the ingredients you have, we've got some great ideas to share with you. Come over to our blog for wholesome recipes and fresh inspiration – nourishbooks.com.